Crib Death

Giulia Ottaviani

Giulia Ottaviani

Crib Death

Sudden Unexplained Death of Infants – The Pathologist's Viewpoint

With 64 Figures and 1 Table

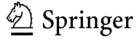 Springer

GIULIA OTTAVIANI, MD
Ricercatore confermato, Professore aggregato
Institute of Pathology, University of Milan
Via della Commenda, 19
20122 Milan, Italy

Tel.: +39-02-50320822; Fax: +39-02-50320823
E-mail: giulia.ottaviani@unimi.it
URL: http://users.unimi.it/~pathol/pathol_e.html

Library of Congress Control Number: 2007921195

ISBN   978-3-540-49370-9   Springer Berlin Heidelberg New York

Springer-Verlag is a part of Springer Science+Business Media
springer.com

Editor: Gabriele M. Schröder Heidelberg, Germany
Desk Editor: Ellen Blasig, Heidelberg, Germany
Cover design: Frido Steinen-Broo, eStudio Calamar, Spain
Typesetting and Production: LE-TEX Jelonek, Schmidt & Vöckler GbR, Leipzig, Germany

Printed on acid-free paper   24/3180/YL   5 4 3 2 1 0

A voice is heard in Ramah, mourning and great weeping, Rachel weeping for her children and refusing to be comforted, because her children are no more.
(Jeremiah 31:15)

To the memory of my beloved mother, Angela,
my first inspiration, and to all parents whose lives
are touched by the tragedy of a child's illness or loss.

Foreword

Thomas N. James

This new book written by Dr. Giulia Ottaviani is beautifully organized and so well written that it is a genuine pleasure to read. It is enjoyable from both an intellectual and a scientific standpoint. I believe it to be a major contribution, not only to "pathology" as she modestly indicates in the title, but to almost every field of medicine, or to anyone with an intellectual curiosity. But for any special medical discipline it could be a virtual necessity. It should be readily available at locations where medical emergency treatment is necessary, especially in hospital emergency rooms and for ambulance medical services.

Pediatricians, obstetricians, and emergency room nurses will find it enormously valuable. It will also be indispensable in numerous other specialties, particularly cardiology, neurology, and even cardiac surgery. For some particular diseases (such as the long QT syndrome) this book will become essential reading, in part because infants, children, and adults can progress to sudden death with this disease.

Very few could have written this book from the standpoint of cardiology and neurology to explain crib death, but I believe that Dr. Ottaviani is uniquely qualified for this mission.

Thomas N. James, MD, MACP
Former Chairman of Medicine and Physician in Chief
at the University of Alabama Medical School in Birmingham
Later, President University of Texas Medical Branch (1987–1997)
Currently Distinguished Professor Emeritus
University of Alabama in Birmingham

Foreword

Luigi Matturri

Infant and perinatal mortality is the most accurate index for evaluating the quality of health in most developed countries. In particular, the fetal mortality rate represents the main indicator of the effectiveness of mother–infant support.

Crib death, or sudden infant death syndrome (SIDS), strikes an apparently healthy baby every 750–1,000 live births and it is the most frequent natural cause of death in the first year of life. The unexpected death of the near-term fetus and of the newborn in the first week of life is unexplained in 60–80% of cases, even after performing a routine post-mortem examination. Data from the World Health Organization indicate that fetal death has an incidence of one in every 100–200 pregnancies in developed countries. Its frequency is therefore six to seven times greater than that of SIDS, and has not significantly decreased during recent years, mainly because of limited research activity.

The results of in-depth investigations performed at the Institute of Pathology of the University of Milan have contributed to the identification of the nature and location of the alterations, common to both SIDS and fetal death, underlying the onset of lethal nervous reflexes. They are mostly congenital anomalies of the vegetative nervous system and/or of the cardiac conduction system, i.e. of the electric switchboard of the heart, which is also under the control of the autonomic nervous system.

Italian Law no. 31 of 2 February 2006 "Regulations for Diagnostic Post Mortem Investigation in Victims of Sudden Infant Death Syndrome (SIDS) and unexpected fetal death" represents a milestone in health politics. It is new and revolutionary and states fundamental rules to significantly reduce the toll in human life: the promotion of anatomoclinical, genetic and epidemiological research, and awareness and information campaigns, and the implementation of programs and projects for the psychological support of victims' families.

The need to submit these small victims to post-mortem examination and to accurate histological investigations is unanimously recognized. Prevention is mainly based on the recognition of lesions detectable in various organs, particularly of the autonomic nervous system regulating the vital activities (respiratory, cardiac, digestive and arousal) and of the pathogenic role of the major risk factors (cigarette smoking and maternal alcoholism, air pollution, sedatives, etc.)

Being a problem of high scientific complexity, the law enacts rules for the post-mortem procedures, with the necessary parents' consent, and it establishes criteria to identify local reference centers, with recognized professional and scientific competences, according to the diagnostic guidelines devised by the Institute of Pathology of the University of Milan.

In the present book a systematic study is presented of the autonomic nervous system and cardiac conduction system in a large number of infants and fetuses dying suddenly and unexpectedly, as well as in age-matched control cases. The purpose of this book is to describe the nervous and cardiac histopathological findings and to describe an investigated standardized post-mortem protocol to apply to all cases of sudden unexpected infant and perinatal death.

I wish this monograph all the success it deserves. The book is aimed at pathologists, neonatologists, pediatricians and researchers with a university degree in medicine or biology, laboratory histotechnicians, pediatric nurses, as well as medical students and general practitioners. I am sure that the readers will be able to learn from it useful tools and hints to apply in their research and practice.

Luigi Matturri, MD
Full Professor of Pathology
Chairman, Institute of Pathology
University of Milan

Preface

This book is based on my PhD dissertation defended at the University of Milan on 3 February 2004.

The sudden unexpected death of a baby in the crib is surely one of the most heartbreaking tragedies for the family and for society. Everyone who reads this book has always to keep in mind that crib death is the leading form of death in otherwise healthy babies within the first year of life. Most of the people and even physicians underestimate the frequency of this problem and do not know how devastating its consequences are. The sudden unexpected death of a baby is so out of order with the sequence of life that there has been no preparation. The parents' terrible loss is then compounded by feelings of guilt; they blame themselves for overlooking possible baby's symptoms or signs. Poignantly and most sadly, the death occurs too often when no one is around, with the dead infant only being discovered later.

After an unexpected sudden infant death a post-mortem examination will be performed. This involves examination of the body, organs and tissues by a pathologist. In this monograph I present a systematic study of the cardiac conduction system and of the autonomic nervous system carried out in a large number of cases.

There is a point that I wish to clarify. The term SIDS (sudden infant death syndrome) is a mistake. It takes origin from its popularization by people who did not know the anatomopathological basis of this form of death. The correct term is sudden death of a baby or infant, crib death (in the United States) or cot death (in the United Kingdom). SIDS is an abhorrent term to families and physicians who care for these tragic cases. Unfortunately, it is also often quoted in my monographs, and I apologize for the use of this terminology.

I wish to transmit to readers the interesting and expanding knowledge of the pathology of crib death and to make them aware of the important role and viewpoint of the pathologist.

Giulia Ottaviani

Acknowledgments

I am very grateful to Prof. Luigi Matturri, MD, Chairman, and to Prof. Anna Maria Lavezzi, MD, Associate Professor, of the Institute of Pathology, University of Milan, for heartily encouraging me to pursue academic research on the pathology of sudden infant and perinatal death. Their valuable support and teaching made this book possible. Sincere thanks are given to Prof. Thomas N. James, MD, MACP, University of Texas Medical Branch at Galveston, for guidance and help. I pay respectful tribute to the memory of Prof. Lino Rossi, MD, Honorary Fellow, American Heart Association Council on Clinical Cardiology, a valued and much appreciated teacher. Appreciation is extended to the staff histotechnicians, particularly Dr. Graziella Alfonsi for skillful assistance. Finally, I am indebted to Prof. Simone Gusmão Ramos, MD, PhD, University of São Paulo, for encouraging this research from the early years of my residency in pathology.

Contents

Introduction and Aims

Now two prostitutes came to the King and stood before him. One of them said: "My Lord, this woman and I live in the same house. I had a baby while she was there with me. The third day after my child was born, this woman also had a baby. We were alone; there was none in the house but the two of us. During the night this woman's son died because she overlaid on him. (1 Kings 3:16–19)

The sudden and unexpected death of a young baby is surely one of the most emotional tragedies that any parent can experience. An understandable continued and growing concern has led to a search for an explanation with the goal of being able to either predict or quickly diagnose the infant or term fetus.

Crib death or sudden infant death syndrome (SIDS) is defined as the sudden death of an infant under one year of age which remains unexplained after a thorough case investigation, including performance of a complete autopsy, examination of the death scene, and a review of the clinical history [280]. Crib death is the most frequent form of death during the first year of life, striking one baby in every 700–1,000 [35]. The emotional consequences among families are devastating, and the social cost is high, especially considering the early loss of many potentially productive individuals [26]. Poignantly and perhaps most sadly, the death occurs too often when no-one is around, with the dead baby only being discovered later. SIDS represents a great enigma as one of the main open issues in the social–medical and scientific setting of modern medicine. Despite a wide spectrum of proposed theories, its etiology remains uncertain.

The most important pathogenetic theories in SIDS are the respiratory (apnea), the cardiac (arrhythmogenic), and the visceral dyskinetic (glottic spasm and/or esophagogastric reflux) theories [76, 77, 239]. It has been stressed that neurogenic factors play a role in all these theories, but particularly in the cardiac arrhythmogenic one since the cardiac conduction system and the accessory pathways are strictly controlled by the autonomic nervous system (respiratory, cardiovascular, and upper digestive) [58, 73, 118, 133, 163, 167, 181, 238].

There is an association between SIDS and sleep, and there are data indicating impaired autonomic function in infants who subsequently die of SIDS, or suffer apparent life-threatening events (ALTE) [73, 76, 118]. Pathologically SIDS can be included in the extended domain of neonatal pathology, particularly if within the diagnosis of SIDS one wishes to include the "borderline" SIDS as not definitely separable from the unifying concept of the syndrome.

Sudden intrauterine unexplained death (SIUD) is late fetal death before complete expulsion or removal of the fetus from the mother [115]. Advances in maternal and fetal care have produced a significant reduction in perinatal mortality, but have not changed the prevalence of SIUD. About one-half of perinatal mortalities are the result of SIUD, with a prevalence of 5–12 per 1,000 births [1, 253]; its etiology is largely unexplained. Our studies performed on a large number of cases indicate that a cardiorespiratory (namely respiratory–reflexogenic) pathology, due to minute lesions of the central nervous system (particularly of the brainstem, the site of confluence of the vagosympathetic reflexes), should be considered significant, together with the involvement of the cardiac nervous and conduction system, lamentably often overlooked in autopsy protocols [178].

In this book we review the systematic study of the autonomic nervous system and cardiac conduction system performed in a large number of infants and fetuses dying suddenly and unexpectedly, as well as in age-matched control infants. The cardiac and neuropathological findings are described. The relationship between SIDS and SIUD are also discussed. The purpose of this book is to review all the possible morphological bases of SIDS and to propose standardized investigational studies to be performed in an autopsy protocol to be applied to all cases of sudden unexpected infant and perinatal death.

I.1   Sudden Infant Death Syndrome

I.1.1   Definition and History of SIDS

SIDS is defined as "the sudden death of an infant under one year of age which remains unexplained after a through case investigation, including performance of a complete autopsy, examination of the death scene, and review of the clinical history" [280].

The initial definition of SIDS including the phrases "unexpected by history" and "unexplained after thorough postmortem examination" [280] is under review. In the pediatric literature, "sudden infant death syndrome" is attributed to multiple causes, and therefore cannot be characterized by a unifying etiological concept. Furthermore, the term "syndrome" (i.e. the simultaneous manifestation of preliminary and/or terminal symptoms) does not seem appropriate, since neither the variety of symptoms nor the microscopic aspects justify such a term [238].

Our group has suggested that the current definition of SIDS as "the sudden death of an infant under one year of age which remains unexplained after a thorough case investigation, including performance of a complete autopsy, examination of the death scene, and review of the clinical history" should be modified by the addition of "complete autopsy examination with an in-depth histopathological analysis of the autonomic nervous system and of the cardiac conduction system that can only be entrusted to experienced reliable pathologists" [166].

Historically the aim of investigations into the cause of SIDS was to seek out a potential single cause that could then be held responsible for all cases that occurred [30]. The earliest representation of SIDS is a sculpture dating to 250 A.D. showing the nutrix Severina looking at an infant dead in the crib (Cologne museum, Germany) (Fig. I.1). The Bible (1 Kings 3:16–19) records an infant brought to King Solomon dead as a result of being "overlaid". Originally, It was assumed the infant died as the result of a neglectful mother lying on him. In early history, a mother whose child died of overlaying was punished. In Egypt, about the time of King Solomon, mothers judged responsible for overlaying were condemned to hug the infant for three days and nights as punishment for their neglect [30, 73]. In the 17th century in Sweden, a mother whose child had died was judged by the church. If the church found the mother guilty of overlaying, she was placed in a pillory in front of the church and lost her standing in the church and community. After a public confession, she could be reinstated into the church and community [30, 73]. Later after cribs and cradles had been invented, the idea of accidental overlaying was gradually abandoned. The diagnosis of overlaying could not be applied to an infant that had died in a separate bed from the mother. The diagnosis was changed to crib death or cot death [225].

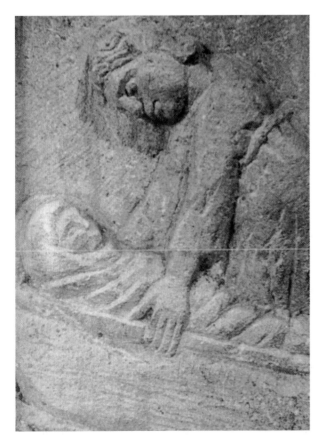

Fig. I.1 The earliest representation of SIDS is this sculpture dating to 250 A.D. which can be seen at the Cologne museum. The nutrix Severina is looking at an infant dead in the crib. This image is adopted as the symbol of the "Lino Rossi" Research Center for the study and prevention of the unexpected perinatal death (of term fetus -stillbirth- and neonatal) and SIDS, University of Milan, Italy

In the 20th century it was found upon autopsy that victims of crib death had an enlarged thymus gland when compared to infants that had died of a chronic disease. At the time, it was thought an enlarged thymus could impinge upon the trachea during sleep resulting in death [30, 73]. In 1923 sleep apnea was first suggested as a cause of crib death. An apnea monitor was recommended to detect and prevent crib death. At the time, an apnea monitor consisted of round-the-clock observation by a trained medical professional [30, 73].

In the 1940s the trend of attributing unexplained infant deaths to status thymico-lymphaticus was decreasing. Instead, these deaths were diagnosed as suffocation by bed linen or posture. The diagnosis of suffocation was based on the assumption that petechiae noted in the thoracic cavity upon post-mortem examination could only have resulted from the act of suffocation [30, 73]. This idea received criticism as it did not explain why a weaker infant (less than 28 days) had a lower incidence of crib death than a larger infant (28 days to 6 months). It was supposed by critics that an older infant was more mobile and less likely to be trapped in bedding than a smaller weaker infant and, therefore, was less likely to be suffocated while sleeping [225]. Additionally, petechiae were not present in all SIDS infants [40].

In 1956 the first epidemiological report on crib death was published. The report stated that certain groups of infants were more likely to be victims of crib death. These included male infants, black infants, premature infants, and infants with a history of upper respiratory infection within the ten days prior to death. Additionally, this report ruled out low levels of gamma globulins as a predisposing factor for infant infection [30, 73, 225].

In 1963 the first international conference on SIDS was held in Seattle, Washington. New findings were presented at the conference. Statistics were presented showing that SIDS also occurs in higher socioeconomic groups, in any sleeping position and while awake, and that 31% of victims were born premature and many were underweight. It was also concluded that any relationship of SIDS to a virus was non-specific, as viral isolation had been done successfully in only one-quarter of all cases [30, 40, 73].

In 1969 the second international conference on SIDS was held in Seattle. At this conference an updated definition of SIDS was agreed upon. Sleep apnea was put to the conference as a possible cause of SIDS, and apnea monitoring was suggested to prevent these deaths. Also presented at the conference was the idea that SIDS was the result of a general vulnerability and combined immaturity interacting with co-incidental additional less-common events [30, 40, 73, 225]. This idea of interacting events as a cause of SIDS was termed the "multifactorial theory" [225].

In 1970 a symposium was held on sudden and unexpected deaths in infancy in Cambridge, UK. At this conference emerged the idea that somewhere there should be a "near miss" form of SIDS [30, 40, 73].

In 1974 a conference on SIDS was held in Toronto, Canada. At this conference it was agreed that the retention of brown fat in the periadrenal area is the result of hypoxia. This retention in some cases was considered possibly due to exposure of the infant to cigarette smoke. It was further determined that the primary problem in SIDS is the failure of the infant to rouse after an apnea event. It was thought that an infant less than one month old has enough remaining anaerobic metabolism after birth to survive an apnea event. It was also thought at this time that an older infant has a decrease in anaerobic metabolism resulting in a decreased ability to survive an apnea event. Additionally, failure to keep the initial follow-up appointment after hospital discharge was associated with a higher rate of SIDS [30, 73, 225].

In 1989 the National Institute of Child Health and Human Development panel redefined the definition of SIDS requiring that the death scene be examined before a diagnosis of SIDS can be made. This addition to the definition of SIDS has been adopted in the United States [225, 280].

In 1992 prone sleeping was shown to be a significant risk factor for SIDS. At this time, the American Academy of Pediatrics (AAP) recommended that infants should be placed on their back to sleep [30, 73, 225]. In 1994 the AAP launched the "back to sleep campaign" [30, 73, 225]. Smoking was again associated with SIDS when elevated levels of nicotine were measured in some SIDS victim's pericardial fluid [30, 73, 225]. The triple risk model was presented by Filiano and Kinney. This states that SIDS results from the interaction of three overlapping factors: (1) vulnerable infant, (2) critical developmental time period in homeostatic control, and (3) exogenous stressor(s) [59]. This approach abandons the tradition of "single cause" research, and instead concentrates on developing an overall understanding of the complexities of infant physiological and pathological responses to a variety of intrinsic and extrinsic factors [30].

I.1.2 Epidemiology and Risk Factors

In countries with reliable epidemiological data (for example, USA, Australia, New Zealand), the incidence of SIDS is almost 1–2‰, striking one in every 700–1,000 otherwise healthy babies [35, 117]. SIDS occurs within the first year of life, with a maximum incidence in the first 6 months of life and a peak incidence from the 2nd to the 4th month [86, 185].

Death generally occurs during sleep, almost always at night between 10 p.m. and 7 a.m. [80]. SIDS is more frequent in males [188], in twins [113], in premature infants [80, 149] and in infants with a low weight at birth [23]. SIDS is more frequent during the winter months and in urban areas [123], in children exposed to thermal stress [219, 252], and in families with a low economic level [9]. The mothers of SIDS infants more frequently are young and unmarried [9] and have more children [9, 80] with a short interval between pregnancies [261], and are more frequently smokers [122, 257], drug addicts [54] or alcoholics [257]. SIDS infants are more frequently the sibling of an infant that previously died of SIDS [80]. Most SIDS victims suffered from infection of the upper respiratory pathways [60, 153] (Table I.1).

The parents of a SIDS infant, besides suffering the obvious emotional consequences of the loss of a child [26, 275], also face problems of a juridical nature, as they are immediately questioned to determine whether they provoked the death of their own child [17]. Besides the psychological trauma from the loss of a child [275], the judicial investigation and forensic autopsy is often the cause of additional suffering.

Table I.1 Risk factors for SIDS. None of the risk factors identified can be considered a specific cause of SIDS. They can be arbitrarily subdivided into amenable and non-amenable to prevention. Modified from Prof. Warren G. Guntheroth, MD, University of Washington School of Medicine, Seattle [74]

Risk factors		Preventive interventions
Amenable	Cigarette smoking by parents	Stop smoking
	Substance-abusing mother	Diagnosis and treatment
	Formula feeding (disputed)	Breast feeding
	Hypoxia in premature infants	Oxygen supplementation at home
	Infections, particularly respiratory	Infant isolation, hygiene, maternal education
	Short interpregnancy interval	Pregnancy interval >6 months
	Pacifiers during the first month if breast-fed	Use pacifiers, particularly if bottle-fed
	No prenatal care	Early prenatal care
	Prolonged apnea, ALTE, near-miss	Work-up, home monitoring
	Poverty, uneducated mother	Education, better housing
	Sleep-related	
	Bed sharing	Cot in bedroom
	Pillows in bed	Avoid
	Prone position in the cot	Supine sleeping position
	Sleeping in separate rooms	Cot in bedroom
	Thermal stress-related	
	Head covered	Avoid duvets
	Room heated	Avoid excessive heating
Non-amenable	Male sex	
	Age (rare after 6 months)	
	Winter	
	Prematurity	
	Sleep	

Much attention has been given to the position of the infant in the crib. Numerous authors [75, 152, 194, 250, 281] state that the prone position is an important risk factor for SIDS. Thus in many countries a campaign has been conducted to encourage mothers to place babies to sleep on their back [152, 194]. Investigations have been carried out to identify the possible risk represented by the type of mattress, bedding, and pillows [111, 187, 266]. Many cases previously recorded as cot death have been proven to be infanticide [218]. The prevalence of non-natural causes of death in babies recorded as SIDS has led to the view that every unexpected infant death should be considered as homicide until proven otherwise [52].

Risk factors associated with a higher risk of SIDS mortality are not claimed to have a causal relationship with SIDS, but have shown a positive statistical relationship. Such factors include the following:

- Prone sleeping position. Of all exogenous stressors identified as associated with SIDS, only one, prone sleeping position, has been shown in studies to significantly reduce the risk for SIDS in healthy full-term infants when eliminated. It is recommended that an infant be placed on its back to sleep [27, 61, 62, 110].
- Soft sleep surfaces and loose bedding. Studies have shown that SIDS is associated with a higher incidence of soft and loose bedding. One proposed mechanism for this is the rebreathing of exhaled carbon dioxide [27, 192]. Additional studies have shown evidence contrary to the rebreathing theory: in countries where infants are routinely placed on sheepskin to sleep there is a negative association with SIDS [30, 73]. Avoiding the use of soft sleep surfaces and limiting the number of loose blankets in the crib may reduce this risk.
- Overheating of the infant. The increased risk of SIDS associated with overheating has been attributed to sleep position, room temperature, excess bedding and infection. A strong association between thermal regulation and ventilatory control has been demonstrated in infants and is thought to play a role in certain cases. Infants that are loosely covered without restricting evaporation do not appear to have as high a risk of SIDS [78].
- Cigarette smoke. A high incidence of SIDS has been associated with exposure to cigarette smoke [12, 27, 192]. Exposure to cigarette smoke in utero has been shown to adversely affect the infant's neural development, and this may provide an explanation. If the parent stops smoking, the risk is decreased [78, 192].
- Bed sharing. Bed sharing with a parent has been associated with an increased risk of SIDS in high-risk populations. Placing the infant in a crib or bassinet will reduce this risk [27, 33].
- Preterm birth and low birth weight. A higher risk of SIDS has been found in this group of infants. No specific mechanism has been proposed for this relationship. Research has shown a decreased risk when preterm and low birth weight infants are placed on their back to sleep [27, 61].
- Marginal nutrition in utero or after birth. Thiamine and magnesium abnormalities have been reported in SIDS victims. It has been proposed that a deficiency in nutritional intake or an abnormality of metabolism may contribute to these abnormalities [146].
- Season. SIDS is more frequent in the winter months [30, 73].
- Infection. A history of a recent upper respiratory infection has been associated with a higher incidence of SIDS mortality [60].
- Lower socioeconomic status. A higher incidence of SIDS has been associated with a lower socioeconomic status. Overall this group tends to have a higher rate of multiple risk factors. It should be noted that SIDS is not limited only to this socioeconomic group [30, 73].

- Maternal factors. Maternal factors associated with a higher rate of SIDS include: mother's age less than 20 years, short intervals between pregnancies, little or no prenatal care, placental abnormalities, and urinary tract infection during pregnancy [30, 73].
- Drenching night sweats. The increased incidence of night sweats in SIDS infants may be related to an abnormality of brainstem function [78].
- Atmospheric pressure changes. A recent study has shown an increase rate of SIDS mortality following a drop in barometric pressure from high to low [32].
- Race. Nearly one-third of all SIDS deaths in the US occur in Native Americans, Alaskan natives, and African Americans (US Department of Health and Human Services, 2000). Causes may include genetic influences, culture, and socioeconomic influences [61].
- Vaccination. A possible role of hexavalent vaccine in triggering a lethal outcome in a vulnerable infant presenting with hypoplasia of the arcuate nucleus (ARCn) and/or cardiac conduction system abnormalities has been suggested [216].

I.1.3 Etiopathogenesis of SIDS

The etiopathogenesis of SIDS is still an unsolved medical problem. SIDS seems to be a "lethal multifactorial dysfunction" due to something not sufficiently developed or to something working in an anomalous way [238]. In the few cases where it has been possible to observe this catastrophic event, a child in apparently good health mysteriously and suddenly stops breathing without crying and without being excited. Most of the babies before the fatal event show only a mild infection of the upper respiratory pathways [60, 153].

The multifactorial problems in the pathophysiology and clinical presentation of SIDS are the result of a controversial and multifaceted pathology [18]. In order to explain SIDS, several theories have been proposed:

1. The cardiac theory, based on myocardial dysfunction altering the diffusion stimulus. Based on this theory, SIDS is considered as a cardiac arrhythmogenic death – QT long and/or preexcitation with malignant tachycardia, atrioventricular (AV) blocks [87, 95, 198, 201, 210, 236, 246, 254, 263, 269].
2. The respiratory theory, based on respiratory alterations, with episodes of sudden and prolonged apnea [77, 153].
3. The visceral dyskinetic theory, based on alterations in upper digestive pathways (motility abnormalities of the glottis and/or gastroesophageal reflux) [109, 279]

It has been stressed that the autonomic nervous reflexes play a role in all such mechanisms. Thus, the anatomicopathological study must include examination of the autonomic nervous system structures involved in the activities of the respiratory, cardiovascular, upper digestive, and cardiac conduction systems [133, 163, 167, 181, 238].

From the anatomicopathological plan, different findings have been reported as possible causes of SIDS: brainstem abnormalities [121], cardiac conduction system developmental defects [72, 199, 269], immaturity of the paraganglia [222, 223], and hyper- or hypoplasia of the carotid bodies [9, 238]. Recently, much importance has been placed on the autonomic innervation of the heart and respiratory apparatus [118, 155, 171, 239].

I.1.3.1 Reflexogenic SIDS

Overall, the abnormalities of the autonomic nervous and cardiac conduction systems do represent a plausible basis for SIDS being reflexogenic in nature (dive, feigned death, cardio-auditory reflexes, Ondine syndrome) [186, 238].

The reflex mechanism more frequently considered in the etiopathogenesis of SIDS is the "dive" reflex, which seems to persist in humans as an inheritance from diver birds and amphibians. It has been reported that washing the face with cold water or plunging into cold water provokes in humans a cardiac deceleration through the ambiguous and the dorsal vagal nuclei. In individuals with an increased sensitivity, bathing the face with cold water can provoke a cardiac arrest. Some people die of cardiac and respiratory arrest while diving, without evidence of drowning. It seems that some newborns with a developmental defect of these reflexogenic centers, i.e. interacting through the glossopharyngeal or trigeminal nerves, die of apnea following absence of breath [145, 180, 238].

Another reflex that seems to play a role in SIDS is the tonic immobility, known as "feigned death" reflex or "fear paralysis" reflex. Small mammals develop a reflex by which they stop breathing or drastically decrease their heart rate when exposed to the danger of a large carnivore. They instinctively realize that the carnivore does not usually devour carrion. The carotid glomus and sinus in the adult mainly regulate cardiac pulsation. In Los Angeles, the police sought to restrain a suspected criminal by pressing the carotid glomus and the sinus provoking death, and this led to the suspension of the police chief because he had encouraged the maneuver [112, 186, 238].

A violent sudden auditory stimulus has been reported to be able to trigger SIDS. This is termed the "auditory" reflex. About 10% of patients with long QT syndrome fall into syncope as a result of the acoustic reflex which is carried by the vestibular nerve along the lateral lemniscus down to the brainstem centers [238, 268]. Cardiac arrest can also occur as a result of the inhibitory oculocardiac reflex, possibly elicited by a prone sleep position [181].

Another reflex considered in SIDS is the so-called "Ondine's curse" reflex. In German mythology, and in a play by J. Giraudoux, Ondine was a water nymph who placed a curse on her unfaithful human lover which took from him all automatic vital functions. He therefore had to remember to breathe and thus would stop breathing when he fell asleep. The so-called reflex of Ondine's curse seems to play a pathological role in SIDS: the baby while sleeping forgets to breathe [238].

Vagal cardiorespiratory reflexes, if pathological, could lead to SIDS [238]. They represent common instinctive conditionings and are physiologically programmed to maintain life under conditions of danger; for example, the dive reflex is vital in diving birds and in amphibians. It is most likely that even minimal alterations along the neural pathways of the reflex arc could interfere with the triggering and/or the reflexogenic response and thus could transform a paraphysiological action into a lethal event. Cardiac or cardiorespiratory arrest could happen whenever such lesions are located in the centers and in the most delicate and complex brainstem neuronal circuitry [233, 238].

I.1.3.2 SIDS due to Metabolic Impairment

In some rare cases of SIDS a hereditary metabolic defect has been detected. The hypothesis that there is a subgroup of SIDS in which death is due to congenital metabolic defects originated from the autopsy finding, in some SIDS victims, of a massive fatty degeneration of the liver similar to that seen in Reye syndrome [29, 63, 70, 148]. Several studies reported in the literature, particularly from the second half of the 1980s, confirm the validity of this hypothesis, but they are discordant as to what percentage of sudden deaths can be attributed to this metabolic factor. Elevated values, ranging from 5% to 27% reported by some authors, are not in agreement with the findings of most recent studies, which have shown that fewer than 3% of SIDS deaths have a metabolic etiology [148, 233]. Although many metabolic diseases can potentially lead to sudden death, only enzymatic defects associated with serious hypoglycemia (often triggered by a subclinical infection), i.e. defects in gluconeogenesis, glycogen metabolism (glycogenosis type I) and beta-oxidation of fatty acids, seem to play a role [29]. In most cases the symptoms suddenly appear following fasting during infection (usually viral in nature) that seems to increase tissue dependence on fatty acid beta-oxidation as an energy source [29, 63, 148].

Among the enzymatic mitochondrial defects involved in the fatty acid beta-oxidation cycle, deficiency in medium-chain acyl-CoA-dehydrogenase (M-CAD) has the richest documentation as a cause of SIDS [63, 148]. In fasting, the metabolic block leads to an insufficient formation of ketone bodies with a reduction in the availability of alternative energy substrates for the brain and the muscles (including the cardiac muscle). This also leads to accumulation of esterified acyl-CoA-dehydrogenase and consequent hypoketonic hypoglycemia [29, 63,148].

In gluconeogenesis defects one of the key enzymes for the process is missing and it is impossible to build glucose from nonglucidic sources (pyruvic acid, lactic acid, amino acids, etc.). Therefore, following fasting, intermediate glycolysis products accumulate with consequent lactic acidemia and hypoglycemia accompanied by a rapid deterioration in the vital functions. In the case of glucogenosis, SIDS has been reported in association with types Ia, Ib and Ic, that imply a deficit in intrahepatic microsomal glucose-6-phosphatase. The activity of this enzyme also seems to remain absent for a prolonged period in most preterm newborns, a group commonly at higher risk of SIDS. The diagnosis is based on the activity of the hepatic enzyme [29, 148].

I.1.4 "Near Miss" and "ALTE" Episodes

The SIDS baby is generally found dead in the crib without prodromic signs. If the infant is seen in the agonic phase, it can be saved with cardiorespiratory resuscitation maneuvers. In recent years the terms "near SIDS" and "near miss" have been used to indicate babies nearly lost, near to death and "resuscitated" after such an episode. Unfortunately, in most cases the dying baby is discovered when the hypoxia and ischemia have already caused irreversible damage to the central nervous system and the myocardium, and every therapeutic measure is too late [258, 259].

Babies with ALTE, which is characterized by apnea and/or alterations in muscular tone or cutaneous color, are at increased risk of SIDS. An ALTE event is considered an abortive SIDS, and babies experiencing an ALTE are considered at high risk of SIDS [14]. Many such babies could possibly be saved by continuous cardiorespiratory monitoring [41, 262].

I.1.5 SIDS Prevention

Since the etiopathogenetic factors in SIDS are still largely unknown, it is not possible to adopt a therapeutic strategy. The incidence of SIDS can be reduced only through preventive approaches. Cigarette smoking is the most preventable risk factor, and should mandatorily be avoided [138, 185].

Once the drama of the loss of a child to SIDS has passed [275], and the trauma of the consequent judicial investigations has been overcome, the parents ask the family practitioner, the gynecologist or the pediatrician: "Can we have another child? Will he/she have any abnormalities? Will he/she be predisposed to SIDS?" The need to give all necessary information to the parents is self-evident [39]. Although cases of SIDS from congenital metabolic dysfunction are rare [148], most authors consider genetic and metabolic investigations necessary in families with a SIDS victim in the following circumstances:

- The sudden infant death was preceded by prodromic signs suggestive of metabolic disease.
- There is a history of sudden death.
- There is a history of Reye syndrome.
- The autopsy of the young victim disclosed fatty degeneration of the liver or of other tissues.
- There has been more than one case of SIDS in the same family [148].

Using the polymerase chain reaction (PCR) method, it is possible to carry out a prenatal diagnosis of a deficit in M-CAD on the chorial villus [71].

In order to recognize babies with long QT syndrome at increased risk of SIDS, some authors have suggested performing screening electrocardiography in all newborns to evaluate cardiac function [254]. According to the AAP [194], a fundamental way to prevent SIDS is by placing newborns and infants to sleep in the crib on their back (supine position). In recent years the incidence of SIDS has decreased in countries where the health authorities have encouraged families to avoid the prone sleeping position for their babies [152, 250]. Because children of mothers who smoke [122, 257], who are alcoholic [257] or who are drug addicts [54] are at higher risk of SIDS, avoiding the parents' smoke, and abuse of alcohol and drugs helps prevent

SIDS. Since infants exposed to thermal stress are at greater risk of SIDS [219, 252], it is also necessary to avoid covering the baby excessively. The children of mothers with a short interval between one pregnancy and the next are also at a higher risk of SIDS [261], so it would seem that the probability of SIDS could also be reduced by informing mothers on this issue.

The domiciliary use of cardiorespiratory monitoring, largely based on the hypothesis that sleep apnea plays a fundamental role in the etiopathogenesis of SIDS, and that the terminal event in SIDS is considered to be reversible with prompt intervention and appropriate resuscitative maneuvers. Generally, babies with a birth weight lower than 1,500 g, those born of drug addict mothers, and those who have presented with idiopathic ALTE episodes are considered at risk of SIDS [14, 39, 41, 259, 262]. Before monitoring it is necessary to perform all relevant tests to exclude any underlying disease (in ill infants, targeted etiological therapeutic strategies are instituted) and to personalize the monitoring program to follow at home.

"Home monitors" allow respiratory and cardiac parameters to be controlled. The monitors have alarm ranges set on a case-by-case basis and have a memory that allows cardiorespiratory activity to be evaluated. The monitor is generally used during the night and while the baby sleeps, mainly during the first 7–8 months of life. If a crisis occurs, the parents are alerted by the monitor when the crisis starts, and generally the infant needs simple "stimulations" administered by the parents. The parents are trained in the appropriate resuscitative maneuvers [138, 262].

I.2 Sudden Intrauterine Unexplained Death

SIUD is late unexplained fetal death before the complete expulsion or removal of the fetus from the mother [42, 115, 171]. SIUD represent about one-half of perinatal deaths, with a prevalence of 5–12 per 1,000 births [1, 253]. The etiology of SIUD is largely unexplained. Advances in maternal and fetal care have produced a significant reduction in perinatal mortality, but have not changed the prevalence of SIUD.

Recent observations have identified, in both SIDS and SIUD victims, frequent developmental abnormalities in the brainstem, particularly in the ARCn [58, 120, 121, 133, 163]. The ARCn is an important cardiorespiratory center of the ventral medullary surface, characterized by great morphological variability [120, 167]. ARCn hypoplasia, detected in over 50% of SIDS and SIUD victims [163, 164], is of great interest, particularly because of its frequency and pathogenetic implications. Sometimes it is associated with alterations in other brainstem structures, particularly the respiratory reticular formation, the solitary tract nucleus, etc. [182]. It is remarkable, particularly because of the functional consequences, that ARCn hypoplasia may be unilateral and when bilateral may involve only part of the nucleus [164]. All these findings need further study in larger series which should involve examination of the brainstem in serial sections in a complete and standardized way.

I.3 Cardiac Conduction System

The heart is regulated by involuntary rhythmic contractions not produced by nervous impulses. The only role of the cardiac innervation, which is primarily sympathetic in nature, is to modify the cardiac rhythm, accelerating or decelerating it. In the common myocardium (or working myocardium) there is a system of particular muscle fibers, called the specialized myocardium, which produces the impulses for contraction which is propagated to the atrial musculature functionally connecting it to the ventricle. The cardiac conduction system is composed of myocardial fibers modified in structure as well as function in comparison to common fibers. Myocardial fibers have scarce myofibrils, abundant glycogen and are slender or star-shaped. They show an elevated spontaneous frequency of contraction and a high speed of impulse conduction [34].

However, these specific or specialized myocells are morphologically not uniform. In generic descriptions of the conduction system, the term Purkinje tissue is commonly used as synonymous with this specific tissue, but this is an over-simplification. In fact, under the light microscope, human Purkinje cells are often of difficult to recognize, and only those of the left bundle branch (LBB) can generally justifiably be called similar to Purkinje cells. The cytological components of the system have several differences. Such morphological heterogeneity reflects the different physiological characteristics of the specialized conduction myocardium in its various centers, in relation to both its autonomic nature and its conductive role.

In the human heart, the system of conduction (and formation) of the stimulus (Fig. I.2) is generally considered to comprise:

- The sinoatrial node (SAN) or Keith-Flack node
- Internodal pathways (superior, middle, posterior)
- The AV node (AVN) or Aschoff-Tawara node
- The AV bundle or bundle of His (common trunk)
- The bifurcation or bifurcating bundle of His
- The right bundle branch (RBB) and LBB

However, it is to be underlined first that the anatomicohistological junctions between the common trunk and the bifurcation, and between the bifurcation and bundle branches are not well delimited, and second that in many cases there is longitudinal partition of tissue destined to become each of the two bundle branches in the background of the common trunk, much above the actual bifurcation (the dualism of the AV pathway sometimes also including the node); therefore the position of the junction–subjunction is uncertain [227, 236, 241, 245].

I.3.1 Sinoatrial Node

In humans the SAN, or Keith-Flack node [116], is an oval formation (about 0.5×1.5 cm in adults), comprising specialized myocardial fibers with abundant interposition of connective tissue. The node is located in the subepicardium, in the superior third of the crista terminalis, directed along its greater axis, in the back wall

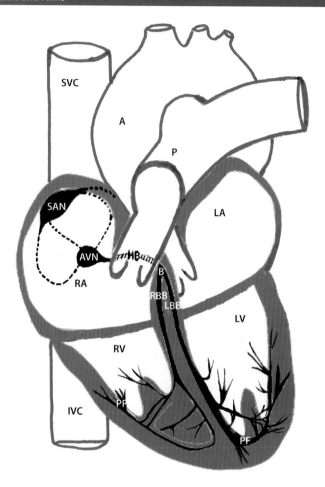

Fig. I.2 Diagram of the human heart showing schematically the location of the cardiac conduction system (A aorta, AVN atrioventricular node, B bifurcation, HB bundle of His, IVC inferior vena cava, LA left atrium, LBB left bundle branch, LV left ventricle, P pulmonary trunk, PF Purkinje fibers, RA right atrium, RBB right bundle branch, RV right ventricle, SAN sinoatrial node, SVC superior vena cava)

of the right atrium. Its cranial part reaches the outlet of the caval vein. The superficial part of the SAN is generally in contact with the subepicardial adipose tissue, while the inner layers variably anastomose with the common atrial myocardium. The SAN artery crosses longitudinally at the center of the SAN (Fig. I.3).

The specialized myocardial cells of the SAN are small (3.0–4.5 μm), clear, with a little evident striation. In the central part of the node the cells weave forming a pluridirectional anastomosis while at the periphery they tend to be parallel and show morphological transitional characteristics towards the adjacent common myocardium. The connective stroma is rich in elastic and reticular fibers close to collagen fibers that, around the SAN artery, tend to have a circular aspect.

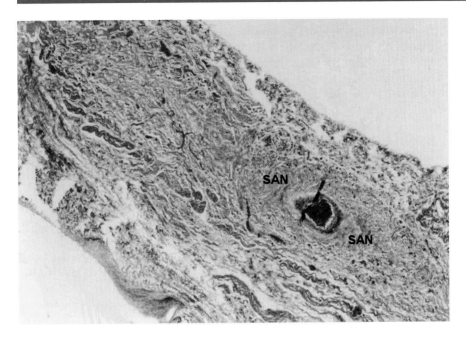

Fig. I.3 Normal human sinoatrial node (SAN) centered by the SAN artery (trichromic Heiden-hain, ×25)

I.3.1.1 Histology

According to James and his school [91], four types of specialized myocardial cells of the SAN can be distinguished:

1. Pacemaker (P) cells, primarily located at the center of the node, rather small and round, assembled in groups with a common basal membrane, characterized by a shortage of myofibrils, sarcosomes and cytoplasmic granules, and by apparent absence of intercalary disks, since the cell–cell contacts are simple juxtaposition of the plasma membranes. In the general organization of the SAN around its artery, the P cells tend to be located centrally [88].
2. Slender cells, rather short and thin, often in relationship with P cells. They are distributed along the whole SAN, but mainly in its external half. Some of these cells extend from the periphery of the SAN for some millimeters into the right atrial myocardium [91]. The slender cells may contain a small or a great number of myofibrils, longitudinally directed (rather than directed randomly as in P cells) with interposition of mitochondria, as in ordinary myocardium. Transitional cells, unlike P cells, contain much glycogen. P cells connect only with each another and with transitional cells, while transitional cells exclusively contact the SAN, as well as the internodal and interatrial tracts. The junctions of Slender cells with P cells are simple, consisting of apposition of the plasma membranes with

many desmosomes, while the junctions among the transitional cells or between these and the cells of the internodal tracts are complex, resembling the ordinary intercalary disks. The framework of these thin fibers is one of the more readily recognizable characteristics of the SAN [88].

3. Common myocardial fibers at the periphery.
4. Purkinje fibers (shorter and wider than the common myocardial cells) with few filaments, with a frayed appearance, clear perinuclear halo, indentations of the sarcolemma in correspondence with the Z stripes. Peculiar to the Purkinje cells is, according to James [91], a "specialized" intercellular junction, an oblique course, constituted by juxtaposition of the plasma membranes, with basal membrane interposition. Also particular to these cells is their rapid myocardial conduction capability, and the lack or paucity of the T-tubular system. Many nerve fibers are intercalated with and adjacent to the nodal cells [65, 157].

Among these specialized types of cells, it is important to recognize the two principal types of cells of the SAN, and it is equally important to understand that the SAN works as a non-elementary biological unit together with three other important anatomic systems: the central artery, the collagen framework, and the innervation [88].

I.3.1.2 Vascular Supply

This is represented by the main atrial artery that lies longitudinally in the SAN. This may originate from the right sinusal nodal artery (deriving from the right coronary artery) in most cases, from the left sinusal nodal artery or from the posterior sinusal nodal artery, deriving from the left coronary artery. Histologically, the SAN artery shows marked development of the longitudinal layer of the tunica media [137, 227, 241]. The normal human SAN is disposed coherently around its homonymous central artery. The SAN has been described as being an enormous adventitia of its artery [88]. The blood introduced into the SAN artery with every cardiac cycle seems to have a modulatory effect. It seems to synchronize the basically random P cell activity stabilizing it from the extranodal influence. Experimental modifications of the pressure of the SAN artery have been shown to have a significant effect on the sinusal pacemaker. This has been further supported by the presence of arrhythmias and sudden death in individuals with anomalous thickness and narrowing of the SAN artery which decrease or eliminate its pulsatility [88].

I.3.1.3 Collagen Framework

After birth, the collagen content of the SAN increases progressively up to adulthood. The growth rate and the final total amount of collagen vary greatly from one human heart to another. The volume of collagen in the adult SAN is so great as to represent the predominant staining feature in histological slides. SAN collagen is a mixture of P cells and slender cells which form a periarterial framework. Furthermore, the collagen separates into small groups of cells, so limiting the extension of cellular contacts. Collagen is an inherent component of both the SAN artery and the basal membrane of the nodal cells. Whatever the exact mechanism by which the central artery influences the pacemaker rate of the SAN, without doubt the normal framework of dense collagen contributes significantly to this functional relationship. Disease damaging the collagen framework is associated with arrhythmias partly due to the loss of this functional relationship and to the consequent instability of the SAN [45]. This suggests that adult individuals with decreased collagen in the SAN could have an intrinsically less stable cardiac pacemaker. If this is the case, then the postnatal development of the fibrous framework of the SAN would play a key role in optimizing the stability of the cardiac pacemaker [88].

I.3.1.4 Innervation

The innervation of the SAN is extremely rich. Numerous and conspicuous nerve trunks reach the SAN, particularly its external surface, through the subepicardial adipose layer where many ganglia (ganglionar plexus) are located. Nerve cells, isolated or in small groups, are sometimes observed in the superficial layers of the SAN. From the perinodal ganglionar plexus, nervous ramifications penetrate the SAN. They seem to form a network with small trunks parallel to the greater nodal axis, gathered by oblique transverse tracts. From this nervous network fascicles or isolated fibers (amyelinated or poorly myelinated) originate with regular swellings or with small variations of caliber to form the preterminal and terminal plexuses [34, 236, 245]. The autonomic innervation influences the SAN and is the principal bond between the normal cardiac pacemaker and the extracardiac regulatory centers, i.e. brain and carotid sinus [88].

In the human heart, both the SAN and the AVN are the two most efficient pacemaker units, the SAN normally being predominant. This predominance is partly due to the more elevated speed and partly to its pacemaker signal distribution pathway to the atria and ventricles, to its abundant adrenergic and cholinergic innervation, and to its disproportionately wide central artery around which the SAN is located in a background of dense collagen [88].

I.3.2 Internodal and Interatrial Pathways

Myocardial fascicles in the right atrium connecting the SAN with the AVN have been described by several researchers. They are: the anterior internodal Bachmann-James tract, also including the principal interatrial connection; the middle internodal Wenckeback tract; and the posterior internodal Thorel tract corresponding to the crista terminalis [227, 241, 236, 245]. The anterior and posterior internodal pathways are more developed and more readily detectable than the middle internodal pathway [91]. The area crossed by the three internodal pathways corresponds to the residual primitive sinus venosus [88]. Experience suggests that the presence of these specific internodal pathways is uncertain. This is mainly due to the long posterior extension of the SAN that, adjacent to the crista terminalis, is rich in "slender cells" of nodal type [65]. James has emphasized the existence and functional importance of the internodal pathways, and has reported their histological features, both at the light and electron microscopic levels, as characterized by the presence of Purkinje cells, but also by nodal (P cells) and slender cells, which are seen predominantly in the conduction system [101]. Such pathways are not covered or otherwise separated from the adjacent tissue. They are anatomically distinguished, being a continuum of myocardial cells in an area otherwise largely consisting of adipose tissue and collagen [88]. The speed of the internodal pathways is significantly higher than in the common myocardium, although it is lower than in the bundle of His and the bundle branches. Moreover, in the normal human heart there is an internodal pathway connecting the SAN with the left atrium [88].

I.3.3   Atrioventricular Node

The AVN, or Aschoff-Tawara node [265], is an oval structure measuring about $1 \times 3 \times 5$ mm, located in the subendocardium of the right atrium, adherent to the central fibrous body, above the septal surface of the tricuspid valve and anterior to the coronary sinus ostium. The proximal border of the AVN is a region where a network of slender nodal fibers contacts the bigger cells and fibers of the internodal pathways [91]. Its supraanterior, lateral and posteroinferior surfaces receive fibers from the adjacent atrial myocardium. In the adult they are fascicles crossing the adipose tissue and partially embracing the AVN before penetrating it (Fig. I.4). In humans, the dimensions of the AVN and the number and type of the atrionodal connections show a certain variability [91, 227].

I.3.3.1 Histology

The AVN is composed of specialized myocardial cells similar to the cells of the SAN but with a rather smaller volume. Their color is weaker than that of the common atrial fibers and they anastomose through short pluridirectional ramifications to form a three-dimensional net, mixed with a collagen and elastic network. Ultrastructurally, James [91] distinguishes four AVN cell types:

1. P cells (see Sect. I.3.1). These are located mainly in the deepest portion of the AVN. They are fewer number in the AVN than in the SAN.
2. Star cells. These are the predominant cell type in the AVN. They anastomose through short pluridirectional ramifications to form a three-dimensional net, mixed with a collagen and elastic network. In the distal portion of the AVN the specialized fibers tend to become parallel [227]. Some star cells are located in the atrial septum with direct contact with the cells of the internodal pathways [88].

Also detected rarely:
3. Common myocardial cells [227].
4. Purkinje cells, particularly in the periphery of the AVN and in the area between the AVN and the right atrial endocardium [88].

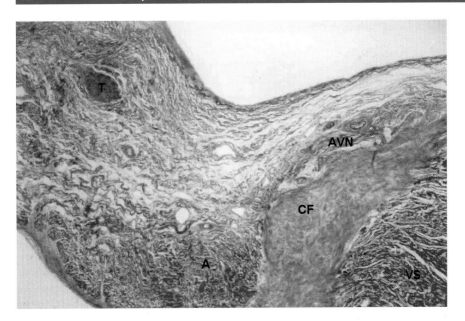

Fig. I.4 Normal human atrioventricular node (AVN). It adheres to the central fibrous body (CF), a dense structure of collagen. The AVN node artery is located eccentrically. The tendon of Todaro (T) is separated from the AVN and located in the right atrium (A), but its location varies greatly in the human heart (VS interventricular septum) (trichromic Heidenhain, ×25)

In the AVN there is much less collagen than in the SAN [88]. It has been suggested that the abundant collagen in the SAN interferes with its pacemaker activity. Therefore, the relatively scanty collagen in the AVN would explain its accessory rather than primary pacemaker role [88].

I.3.3.2 Vascular Supply

The blood to the AVN is assured, in more than 80% of cases, by the branch of the fibrous septum, that is the first perforant septal branch (posterior) of the right coronary artery. The AVN artery (sometimes double or triple) penetrates the node in the inferior posterior portion and crosses it near the center [227]. Unlike in the SAN, in the AVN the homonymous artery is not normally located centrally. The AVN artery is usually eccentric and is often detected out from the node, but almost always it is partly included in the central fibrous body [88]. The AVN artery differs in caliber and in richness of internodal ramifications. It should not be considered a terminal artery, as was previously thought in normal and pathological anatomy. The venous outflow is assured by big channels and sinusoids in the superior part of the node; the veins drain into the coronary sinus or directly into the right atrium [227].

I.3.3.3 Lymphatic Drainage

Lymphatic drainage is assured by a conspicuous system of lymphatic channels originating from the superior portion of the interventricular septum. They reach the cardiac center near the Aschoff-Tawara node.

I.3.3.4 Innervation

Innervation is less relevant in the AVN than in the SAN. However, nerve trunks cross the adipose perinodal tissue and penetrate the node though thin ramifications. Nerve cells have been noted rarely in the human AVN, while some ganglia are readily detected around it, especially in the dog [34, 65, 91, 236, 245].

I.3.4 Morphological Concept of the Atrioventricular Junction

According to the classical description of Tawara [265], which has been little modified over the years, the AVN, the bundle of His, and the two bundle branches represent a myocardial conduction pathway known as the "atrioventricular system" or Tawarian system that is normally the only connection between the atrial and the ventricular myocardium [34, 236, 245].

Electrophysiological studies tended to designate the undivided part of the AVN with its atrial junctions and the bundle of His, up to the bifurcation, by the term of AV junction (AVJ), tissue, or area. This definition which primarily reflects the functional significance, does not offer, from the anatomic point of view, particular advantages in comparison to the traditional nomenclature of the conduction system. Rather, such a definition could lead to a misunderstanding by inferring an incomplete anatomicophysiological continuity of the system itself whose proximal part (undivided) and distal part (divided into two branches) are generally considered to constitute unique entities [34, 227, 236, 241, 245].

The AVJ contains not only the AVN and the bundle of His with its proximal branches, but also the AVN artery (terminal divisions of the septal branches of the anterior descending left coronary artery), the central fibrous body, the tendon of Todaro, the pars membranacea septi, some nerves and ganglia, and the septal surface of both the mitral and tricuspid valves [91]. The origins of both the aorta and the principal pulmonary arteries do not belong to the AVJ, but are adjacent to the AVJ. Being near these mitral and tricuspid valvular surfaces, cardiac contractile movements produce marked stress on the AVJ [91].

The central fibrous body and the tendon of Todaro are two important functional structures for the mechanical strength of the AVJ.

I.3.4.1 Central Fibrous Body

The central fibrous body of the adult human heart is a dense structure of collagen, while in the fetus and in the newborn it is almost entirely a gelatinous substance (Fig. I.4). Based on its mechanical function, the central fibrous body can be described as a septal anchor for the mitral valve, extending directly from the valvular edge to the crest of the interventricular septum where it also provides an attachment for the septal edges of the tricuspid valve. Since both the AVN and the bundle of His lie directly on the central fibrous body, due to their proximity, they are considered at risk in case of alteration to the central fibrous body (for example, in calcification of the mitral ring) [91]. The mitral valve, facing the maximal systolic pressure normally produced by the left ventricle, has a strong influence on the central fibrous body. Therefore, it is also clear why the central fibrous body insertion in the crest of the interventricular septum is rich in fibrous tissue. It is a mistake to think that this fibrous tissue in the crest of the interventricular septum represents a pathological process. Such fibrous tissue is not only normal, but is even necessary to ensure local mechanical strength [91]. The dynamic role played by fibroblasts in the central fibrous body during postnatal morphogenesis of the AVN and the bundle of His has been a matter of controversy [45, 91, 269].

I.3.4.2 Tendon of Todaro

The tendon of Todaro is more prominent in the heart of the dog than in the human heart, in which it is rudimentary. In its typical form (Fig. I.4), the tendon of Todaro originates in the tissue of the atrial septum, anterior to the coronary sinus and well above of the central fibrous body. Rarely it is attached to the wall of the coronary sinus or to the pons of Eustachio. From its origin, it becomes adjacent to the AVN but usually above or separate from it. Then it goes directly to the central fibrous body or, more rarely, to the origin of the aorta [91]. According to its site, which varies greatly in the human heart, it can join the central fibrous body posteriorly adjacent to the coronary sinus or more anteriorly adjacent to the aorta. At both these sites, it can also influence the morphogenesis of the AVN [91].

I.3.5 Bundle of His

The Bundle of His or His bundle (HB) or common trunk is also known as the crus commune. Without any clear histocytological borders with the AVN, it enters the central fibrous body (Fig. I.5). The direction followed by the bundle of His in the central fibrous body is not constant; generally it follows the basis of the central fibrous body on the right side, toward the crest of the interventricular myocardial septum. However, a central location or a location toward the left within the fibrous septum are not rare [227].

The proximal portion of the bundle of His is sometimes distinguished by the penetrating portion entering the fibrous septum. The section of the bundle of His generally has an oval shape, but can vary notably case by case if examined at different levels. The best criteria to establish where the AVN ends and the bundle of His begins and what the AVN includes are still unclear [272]. The origin of the bundle of His can be defined in two different ways. According to the first definition, the bundle of His begins where the AVN becomes separate, through the fibrous body surrounding it, from the atrial septal fibers. According to the second definition, the bundle of His begins where the network of slender cells is connected to the parallel Purkinje fibers oriented

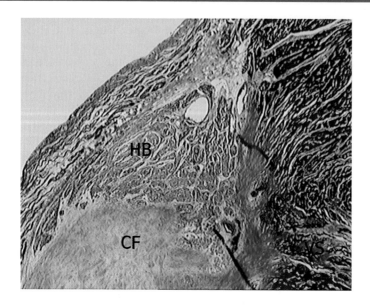

Fig. I.5 Normal human bundle of His (HB) located in the central fibrous body (CF) (VS interventricular septum) (trichromic Heidenhain, ×25)

longitudinally [91]. From the histological point of view, the fibers appear longer and more regularly located than in the AVN. Their caliber is basically uniform, except in the area close to the bifurcation where tortuous and irregular fibers appear. The transverse striation is more evident; the nuclei are smaller. The color remains in general less evident than in the common myocardium. The subdivision of the bundle of His into fibers directed to the two branches, as described by Sciacca et al. [256] in an original way several years ago, has been confirmed in the modern physiopathological concept of the functional dualism in the longitudinal dissociation of the AV pathway, as well as in the "junctional" pathogenesis of the AV blocks [34, 227, 236, 245].

I.3.5.1 Histology

The bundle of His is composed, from its origin, of small nodal fibers of mean cross section 7×5 µm. The fibers gradually increase in diameter and become oriented parallel. James [88] states that the common trunk is mainly composed of Purkinje cells oriented longitudinally and separated by basically continuous collagen septi, with few transverse anastomoses [91].

I.3.5.2 Vascular Supply

Usually the common trunk and the bifurcation are vascularized by arterioles originating from the ramus septi fibrosi (right coronary artery). However, some anatomicoclinical cases have shown that damage to the common trunk has been caused by alterations to the anterior descendant of the left coronary artery [34, 227, 236, 241, 245].

I.3.5.3 Innervation

Small nerves run down along the vessels of the common trunk; they are also observed in the fibrous septum [236, 245].

I.3.6 Bifurcating Bundle of His or Bifurcation

The common trunk bifurcates after having assumed, in frontal section, a markedly more prismatic shape (Fig. I.6). The division is at the level of the interventricular myocardial crest; it is almost never symmetrical and therefore it is observed with difficulty in single histological sections. Usually the bifurcation is located on the right side, the RBB being the continuation of the common trunk. However, in some cases it has been observed on the left side. In single sections, the appearance is characterized by the scarcity of bundles directed to the left compared to those of the RBB. This is not so much due to a great quantity of fibers in the RBB, but due to the fact that the fibers of the LBBs radiate precociously, departing from the common trunk at the single levels as isolated ramifications. The fibers of the RBBs represent instead a compact bundle. An interesting but generally neglected aspect of the Tawarian bifurcation is its variability, in both site and direction. This variability is not a purely anatomic issue, but also seems to play a role in the field of anatomicopathological "vulnerability", with the well-known consequences on atrial and intraventricular conduction. In fact, the bifurcation sometimes does not appear to be located as a "rider" of the ventricular myocardial septal crest, according to the classical description, but on the contrary is located on a side, usually the right side, of the ventricular myocardium. So, as mentioned above, the bifurcation is displaced to the left side and the LBB runs down directly in the left subendocardium, while instead the RBB originates as a bundle included in the septal myocardium. Then the RBB runs an "intramural" course before reaching a subendocardial location. In rare cases the bifurcation is totally intramyocardial. It is located in the ventricular septum, so that both the branches have an intramural origin, and then go towards the respective endocardium [34, 236].

I.3.7 Right Bundle Branch

The RBB (Fig. I.6) appears as the continuation of the common trunk, from which it continues first in a horizontal direction, and after passing under the confluence of the anterior and middle cuspides, passes under the right septal endocardium for about 0.5 cm. It then turns to the lower part and penetrates the muscular septum staying separate from it by a connective fold. After 1 cm it becomes subendocardial again and frays out near the base of the anterior papillary tricuspid muscle. Not rare in humans is the anatomic variant (connected to that described as bifurcation)

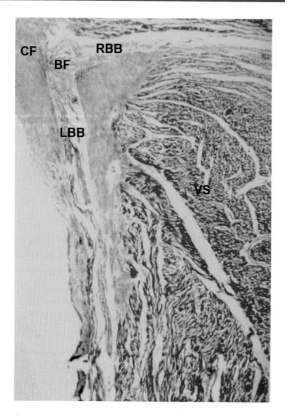

Fig. I.6 Normal human bifurcating bundle of His (BF). The
left bundle branch (LBB) runs
directly down in the left subendocardium, while the right bundle
branch (RBB) originates in the
septal myocardium and has an
intramural course before reaching a subendocardial location
(VS interventricular septum, CF
central fibrous body) (trichromic
Heidenhain, ×25)

where the root of the RBB directly penetrates the interstitium of the septal myocardium, so underlining a first intramural rather than a subendocardial portion. Such a
variant may have anatomicopathological significance if it causes an alteration in the
branch with regional myocardial infarctions leading to direct or indirect compro-
mise through a perifocal inflammatory reaction.

I.3.7.1 Histology

In its upper third the histological features of the RBB are the same as those observed
at the level of the bifurcation. In the middle third it does not show any remarkable
difference compared with the myocardium [34, 227, 236, 241, 245].

I.3.7.2 Vascular Supply

The RBB is fed by a branch of an anterior septal artery (left coronary artery) [236,
245].

I.3.7.3 Innervation

In the RBB there are no macroscopic nerves. Amyelinated fibrils are always detectable close to the myocardial fibers and to the capillaries by electron microscopy [34, 227, 236, 245].

I.3.8 Left Bundle Branch

The LBB (Fig. I.6) arises from the common trunk and is directed toward the homologous side of the ventricular septum as a thin bundle of fibers maintaining along their course a subendocardial location and an appearance similar to Purkinje fibers. A rare intramyocardial variant of the proximal LBB has been recently identified. The LBB 1–2 cm from its origin becomes fan-shaped subdividing in a complex and variable manner into richly and precociously anastomosed ramifications. A frankly dichotomous subdivision of the LBB is rare in the human heart [34, 227, 236, 245].

I.3.8.1 Histology

In the LBB of the human heart there are many cells of Purkinje type [236, 245].

I.3.8.2 Vascular Supply

The anterior and middle ramifications of the LBB, which is broadly located on the left surface of the septum, are vascularized by the anterior perforant arteries (left coronary artery), and the posterior ramifications by the posterior perforant arteries (right coronary artery). Since the anterior perforant arteries are long, they also supply the intermediate area of the LBB. It must be underlined that the LBB, due to its subendocardial location and extension, is also oxygenated trans-endocardially by blood circulating in the ventricle [34, 227, 236, 245].

I.3.8.3 Innervation

In humans the innervation of the LBB is limited, histologically at the light microscopic level, to thin and rare amyelinated subendocardial fibrils. On electronic microscopy, in contrast, the richness of the innervation of the branch is evident. In the guinea-pig heart, nervous amyelinated fibers are composed of two to six protoaxons, each refolded by a mesoaxon (deriving from the invagination of the plasma membrane of the lemnoblast). Such fibers are tightly linked to the sarcolemma of the myocardial cell of the branch, sometimes showing vesicles of the axoplasm of presynaptic cholinergic type [34, 236, 245].

I.3.9 Fetal and Postnatal Development of the Conduction System

The cardiac conduction system, proportionally wider in the fetus, is reduced in the newborn and even more in the adult. It seems that this reduction happens mainly by apoptosis. This is genetically programmed cellular death, not a result of illness, but perhaps secondarily caused by illness [38, 95]. In fact, it seems that developmental alterations in the cardiac conduction system after birth can lead to arrhythmias responsible for sudden and unexpected infant death [22, 89, 91, 150, 198, 200, 205, 263].

I.3.9.1 The Sinoatrial Node: Fetal and Postnatal Development

During the 6th to the 8th gestational week, the heart already shows many of its adult features and the SAN is already detectable. The cells of the SAN originate in the venous sinus. At this early stage, the cells of the SAN are all similar and appear as small dark cells. It seems that these cells are specialized since they arise and develop from primordial pacemaker sites [88].

At around birth, the P cells and the slender cells quickly also become distinguishable on light microscopy, but they are a site of continuous further differentiation during the first years of life [88].

In the adult SAN there are relatively fewer P cells than in the fetus and the newborn, while the slender cells are more frequent in the adult SAN [88].

SAN Artery

During the early stages of fetal development, the SAN already contains a small artery, but its size increases during childhood and adolescence. During fetal development it appears as part of the arterial ring distributed at the junction of the venous sinus and the atrium [88]. Some cells of the developing SAN are able to produce an electric impulse functionally totally independent of the central artery. The sinusal rhythm in the fetus and the newborn is fast and relatively unstable, unlike in the adult where it is slower and much more stable [88].

Collagen Framework

A concomitant and tightly correlated feature during development is the increasing content of collagen. After birth, the collagen content of the SAN increases progressively up to adulthood, but the growth rate and the final amount of collagen vary greatly from one human heart to another. The volume of collagen in the adult SAN is so high as to represent the most readily distinguishable staining feature in histological slides for light microscopy. The postnatal development of the fibrous stroma of the SAN plays a key role in optimizing the stability of the normal cardiac pacemaker [88].

SAN Innervation

Early during fetal development, there is clear evidence of cardiac cholinergic innervation, while adrenergic innervation develops afterwards and is completed only some months after birth [88]. The scarcity of adrenergic innervation of the fetal and neonatal SAN can be compensated for by an increased sensitivity of the SAN to circulating catecholamines. The variability in autonomic influence through intranodal release of neurotransmitters should be one of the most efficient forms of control. The nervous control of the fetal and infant SAN is mainly cholinergic. The balanced autonomic innervation is developed in the postnatal SAN when the SAN has become intrinsically a generator of more stable impulses [88].

I.3.9.2 Internodal Pathways: Fetal and Postnatal Development

Little is known about the fetal and postnatal development and changes in the internodal pathways, although many markers can be seen in the adult since the fetal heart completes its subdivision in the second month of gestation. Since the anterior and middle internodal pathways merge in the interatrial septum and since normally the oval foramen closes shortly after birth, it is probable that the septal course of the internodal pathways becomes well defined only during postnatal life. In cases of anomalous development of the atrial septum or of the primitive venous valves, it can be anticipated that the internodal conduction pathways will be altered [88].

I.3.9.3 Atrioventricular Node Development

During embryonal development, the primitive AVN migrates inside the heart from its original epicardial center when the dorsal endocardial pillow invaginates during formation of the AV valves. The artery supplying the AVN originates from a large vessel that penetrates directly into the interventricular posterior vein near the junction with the coronary sinus. This suggests that the dorsal endocardial pillow migrates to the inside transporting with it the AVN and its artery [88]. Additional evidence for this migration of the AVN to the inside is the onset of mesotheliomas which certainly originate from primitive residual cells incorporated in the primitive heart by the adjacent epithelial tissue during embryonal development [6]. The primitive AVN is thought to originate at the level of the junction of the superior cardinal vein and the venous sinus. Then, with the development of the left atrium and the incorporation of the venous sinus into the atrium, the AVN may move towards its adult location or may remain in the same location while the atria develop around it. The terminal portion of the left superior cardinal vein becomes the coronary sinus, while the proximal portion usually atrophies. In the human embryonic heart, immediately after the first month of gestation, the AVN can already be detected on histological examination. At this stage, it is vaguely organized, but is already in its characteristic location in relation to the central fibrous body that is still gelatinous in consistency [91].

Both the AVN and the bundle of His are modified little or not at all during the remaining fetal life, but within 1 or 2 weeks of birth they undergo dramatic transformation [91].

In the infant heart, there are fragments of nodal AV tissue dispersed along all the borders of the central fibrous body (including the ventricular septal crest). They are gradually reabsorbed during postnatal development, so that they are rarely seen in the adult heart [88].

Postnatal morphogenesis of the AVN and bundle of His is an important part of the normal development of the cardiac conduction system. The term "resorptive degeneration" was originally suggested by James in 1968 [87] to indicate the normal process of postnatal cardiac molding, consisting of degeneration, cell death and replacement in an orderly programmed way [38, 88, 91, 95]. The nature of the changes in the conduction system during the postnatal period and their relationship to sudden death in infancy is still a subject of debate [198, 210].

I.3.9.4 Bundle of His and Bundle Branches Development

It seems that the bundle of His and bundle branches originate in a different way from the AVN. Some factors suggest that the bundle of His and its branches originate separately from the ventricular crest [88]:

1. Mesotheliomas rarely extend beyond the proximal border of the bundle of His, with a predominant location around and inside the AVN.
2. The action potential of the membranes of the cells of the AVN and bundle of His are very different.
3. All cases of congenital AV block studied histologically have basically shown the same lesion: an interruption between the AVN and the bundle of His, despite the presence of both structures.
4. In a clinical–pathological study of the absence of SAN activity and AV block in a dog, the cells of the SAN and of the AVN appeared not to be differentiated in their adult configuration, while the cells of the bundle of His and its proximal branches were normal.
5. The area of the junction between the AVN and the bundle of His appears to be a locus minoris resistentiae from the electrophysiological point of view, and because of its tendency to undergo focal ischemic degeneration, in both humans and dogs.

None of these factors prove in themselves the separate origin of the AVN and the bundle of His, but taken together they strongly suggest this [88].

In the human embryonic heart, soon after the first gestational month, the bundle of His, similarly to the AVN, can be easily distinguished on histological examination. At this stage it is vaguely organized, but it is already in its characteristic site in relation to the central fibrous body that is still gelatinous in consistency [91]. The bundle of His in fetal life differs from its adult configuration in at least two important aspects: it is disproportionately large and wide, and it is widely attached to or in direct continuity with the myocytes of the interventricular septal crest [91]. The AVN and the bundle of His do not change or change little during the remaining fetal life, but within 1 or 2 weeks of birth they undergo some "dramatic" transformations [91].

I.3.9.5 AVN and Bundle of His Postnatal Molding

It has been shown that the human AVN and the bundle of His undergo extensive postnatal molding before reaching their adult configuration [87]. This should not be surprising, there being already many well-known examples of cardiac and great vessel molding after birth (for example, the closure of the oval foramen and the ductus arteriosus) [88].

When the central fibrous body starts to change from a large gelatinous mass to a thin but strong fibrous mass in the adult heart, the AVN and the bundle of His undergo what Grant in 1962 initially defined as a formation and remodeling process [69, 91]. Grant [69] described many postnatal events of the heart, such as the closure of the oval foramen and of the ductus arteriosus, and the thinning of the right ventricle wall. Similarly, the AVN and the bundle of His also undergo a remarkable postnatal transformation [69, 91]. In general terms, this postnatal molding of the AVN and the bundle of His can be considered as a molding and shaping process through which the surplus tissue is gradually reabsorbed so that these two electrically important structures are refined into their adult configuration [91]. Many strands of surplus AVN tissue protruding into the central fibrous body of the fetal heart, the abundant conductive tissue connecting the fetal bundle of His with the ventricular septum, and most of the surplus volume of the bundle of His are reabsorbed [91]. It is interesting that this postnatal reabsorption of the bundle of His in humans takes place exclusively on its left side and never on the right.

The postnatal molding of the AVN and the bundle of His is ubiquitous in all normal hearts. This represents their transformation from a rough configuration, that may be electrically dangerous in the fetus and newborn, into their more smooth, and safe adult configuration [91]. During the molding, the gradual reabsorption of the AVN and bundle of His cells seems to be a genetically programmed process. What begins and finishes the process within the first or second year of life in normal infants is unknown [91]. Inevitably, this process of postnatal morphogenesis is correlated with cellular death [87, 91], but this should be considered normal as many other examples of cellular death are associated with human morphogenesis [251].

The molding of young fibroblasts of the central fibrous body and of young growing cells of the AVN and bundle of His includes cellular death and focal cellular degeneration that can have dangerous consequences [87]. It has been proposed that congenital AV block represents an excessive growth of collagen along the bundle of His, jeopardizing its connection with the AVN. However, since homeostasis between the AVN/bundle of His and the central fibrous body cells is reached only some months or years after birth, the hypothesis of "over development" to explain congenital AV block would require that the block appears initially in the postnatal period, while it is already detectable prenatally. This strongly suggests (but it does not prove) that congenital AV block is due to incomplete development of the junction between the AVN and the bundle of His, rather than to a postjunctional overdevelopment of collagen [91].

Since AVN/bundle of His molding normally does not begin before birth, it can be suggested that postnatal events trigger the process. Hemodynamic cardiac and great vessel modifications at birth could be responsible for this process. If so, then the great physical stress normally involving the central fibrous cardiac body could induce modification of the functional relationship between young fibroblasts located therein and the adjacent AVN/bundle of His cells. There is also the possibility that the AVN/bundle of His cells are subject to genetic control leading to degeneration at a particular time or under particular conditions, as for instance during the postnatal hemodynamic changes. It is uncertain what factors control AVN/bundle of His molding in the postnatal period, but it is certain that the process takes place as one of the most important developmental changes of the cardiac conduction system [88].

I.3.10 Accessory Cardiac Conduction Pathways

Tawara [265], in his original description of the AVN, considered it as the beginning of the bundle of His and therefore the tract through which all the electrical activity of the atria is transmitted to the ventricles. This is true only in normal circumstances [91]. The impulse goes down from the SAN towards the ventricle, stops in the AVN where its speed is 2 cm/s. The point where the impulse passes from the bundle of His to the two bundle branches can be compared to a highway crossroads. In the SAN and in the AVN the impulse slows down, while in the bundle of His it speeds up [236, 245].

At the level of the AVJ there are transmission pathways, both normal and abnormal, in which the AVN can be partially or completely bypassed. A complete bypass of the AVN represents both an anatomic and a physiological abnormality, and it can be both near to or far from the AVN and the bundle of His [91]. When a complete bypass is next to the AVN, the fibers pass from the atrial septum through the central fibrous body independently of the AVN but directly connecting with the bundle of His [91].

In some cases a defective reabsorption of the fetal tissue, perinatal or postnatal, as well as the same "highway", there are also accessory pathways directed toward the ventricles. Such malformations, under a neurovegetative influence, can induce cardiac activity dysfunction leading to cardiac arrhythmias and sudden death [97, 231].

When there is a working accessory AV connection, the whole AV system or its junctional tract, can become part of the classic circuit of a tachycardic macroloop. It is well known that preexcitation depends on the presence of AV accessory pathways where the impulse can diffuse in an antegrade direction [181, 228].

The AV accessory connections are divided in three principal categories:

1. Direct accessory pathways, completely connecting the atrium to the ventricle through the conduction system (Kent fibers). They are subdivided into right, left, and medial.
2. Indirect accessory pathways, connecting the atrium to the ventricle through an anatomicofunctional interposition of junctional tissue. They are subdivided into:
   - mediate pathways for distal "input" within the cardiac conduction system, known as atriofascicular James fibers. They come down from the atrium and enter the junctional area beyond the nodal AV site of impulse deceleration.
   - mediate pathways for "output", known as Mahaim fibers. They originate from the AVN, from the bundle of His and/or from the bifurcation and anastomose early with the septal ventricular myocardium. These mediate emission bun-

dles of the Mahaim type, and are subdivided into superior (nodoventricular), middle (fascicular-ventricular) and inferior (ventricular bifurcation).
3. Mixed accessory pathways, direct and indirect. They are represented by Kent medial and Mahaim superior pathways [181, 228, 231].

While the Kent-type direct bundles can be found anywhere on the contour of the AV rings (mostly on the subepicardial area) and in the region of the trigonum (defective in such cases), James and Mahaim fibers are always located in the junctional area. The presence of AV accessory pathways is the necessary, but not sufficient, condition to determine preexcitation and/or reciprocating tachyarrhythmias. Such arrhythmias can start or stop depending on their uni- or bidirectional conductive activity under neurovegetative control [97, 228, 231]. Embryology suggests that such anomalous connections represent the vestiges of the incomplete separation of the cardiac conduction system from the adjacent myocardium, and/or of the primordial mixture of atrial and ventricular myocardium in the fetal, newborn or infant heart. In fact, anomalous AV pathways are not rare. The malformations of accessory and/or double AV pathways have two possible causes. First, there may be defective reabsorption and shaping of the junctional tissue in the pre- and postnatal period, when the so-called "archipelago" of specific myocardial islands constituting the AVN/bundle of His axis should partly degenerate at the periphery and reunite in the mature AVJ. Second, there may be defective development of the AV fibrous rings and of the central fibrous body. This frequently seems to occur concomitantly with a low insertion of the medial tricuspid leaflet, so configuring a cardiac malformation microscopically similar to Ebstein disease called "micro-Ebstein" malformation. This micro-Ebstein malformation is characterized by a narrow muscular septum–septal connection composed of a direct mediate Kent bundle, mediate Mahaim fibers, or both the accessory AV pathway types [228, 231, 236].

I.3.10.1 Kent Fibers

The Kent fiber is an accessory direct arrhythmogenic pathway. It connects the atrium with the ventricle bypassing the classical conduction system. This anatomic defect results in double conductive pathways, with an accessory conduction pathway that does not slow down in the AVN. This represents the anatomic substrate for the ventricular preexcitation syndrome or Wolff-Parkinson-White (WPW) syndrome. The Kent bundle allows the passage of a faster impulse than the normal pathway because the deceleration in the AVN is skipped. A tachycardic preexcitation of the ventricle, and the possibility of retrograde excitation of the atrium through the Kent bundle follow. The impulse through the Kent bundle enters directly into the ventricle and can reenter along the septum crossing the conduction system in a retrograde way. The anomalous flow of reentry can cause a sudden ventricular fibrillation [236, 245].

Direct Kent fibers have been described in over 60% of patients with WPW syndrome who show a short P–Q time and delta wave. The pathogenetic role of the Kent bundle is confirmed by remission of preexcitation malignant arrhythmias after resection of the anomalous bundle [228, 243].

I.3.10.2 James and Mahaim Fibers

These are bundles directly connecting the atrial common myocardium to the specific myocardium (AVN, bundle of His or bifurcation). James fibers are atriofascicular accessory pathways connecting the atrium with the bundle of His. Unlike the Kent bundle, the pathogenetic significance of the mediate bundles of James and Mahaim type is unclear, both in relation to the Lown-Ganong-Levine (LGL) syndrome without delta wave due to atriofascicular fibers, or to the P–Q variant WPW syndrome with delta wave due to nodo- and fasciculoventricular Mahaim fibers [193, 244].

I.4   Central, Peripheral and Autonomic Nervous Systems

The regulation of cardiac rhythm is hardly distinguishable from that of vessel motility and respiratory activity, both from the anatomic and the physiological points of view. The neurovegetative innervation, cardiovascular and respiratory, comprises the central structures (nuclei of the brainstem and of the spinal cord) and the peripheral receptors, together with the nerves and ganglia. They are part of the mechano- or baroreceptor reflex arc that, with particular superior psychoemotional integrations, seems to condition dysfunctions of varied intensity and sudden reflex death [181, 178].

The nervous control of the heart is due to the antagonism between sympathetic and vagal innervation. The central parasympathetic nuclei are situated in the brainstem while those of the sympathetic nervous system are located in the thoracic spinal cord [181, 178].

I.4.1   Brainstem

The nuclei that regulate cardiovascular and respiratory activities are located In the floor of the fourth ventricle, in proximity to the obex. In humans the two principal vagal visceromotor nuclei are located above the ependyma: they are the dorsal vagal nucleus and the ambiguous nucleus [181, 178].

I.4.1.1 Arcuate Nucleus

The ARCn is located in the ventral surface of the medulla, close to the pyramidal bundles, and it extends longitudinally from the caudal border of the pons to the inferior pole of the olive. The neurons, which are polygonal or oval in shape, have average dimensions. The ARCn plays an important role in chemoreception, modifying blood gas exchange (oxygen and carbon dioxide) and acidity. The neuronal circuits of this vital area of the brainstem elaborate afferent and efferent stimuli, integrating both with impulses of the sympathetic thoracocervical chain, and with corticomesencephalic psychosensorial descending impulses. The reflexogenic reply is carried particularly along the motor fibers of the dorsal vagal nucleus. It is well known that barochemoreptorial reflexogenesis changes the cardiovascular vagal-sympathetic equilibrium in favor of the first (bradycardia, vasodilatation). However, in pathological cases with neurovegetative impairment, an altered vagal response may predispose to a violent sympathetic predominance (tachycardia, hypertension), lowering the threshold of ventricular fibrillation, leading to a high risk of sudden death. Moreover, the receptors are activated by circulating catecholamines [181, 178].

I.4.1.2 Parabrachial/Kölliker-Fuse Complex

The parabrachial/Kölliker-fuse (PB/KF) complex is a pontine complex which plays an important role in modulating respiratory function. Morphologically, the PB/KF complex has been described as a group of neurons that surrounds the superior cerebellar peduncle, subdivided into three well-defined regions:

1. The medial parabrachial nucleus, localized ventromedially to the superior cerebellar peduncle.
2. The lateral parabrachial nucleus, located dorsally to the superior cerebellar peduncle.
3. The Kölliker-Fuse (KF) nucleus, located ventrally to the lateral parabrachial nucleus.

The complex has inhibitory activity, temporary during fetal life, acting on chemoreceptor function and particularly on the pulmonary motor responses to blood changes in pO_2, pCO_2, and pH. After birth the structures of the PB/KF complex participate in modulation of respiratory activity [36, 82, 136, 193].

I.4.1.3 Dorsal Motor Vagal Nucleus

The dorsal motor vagal nucleus consists of neurons of average size. It contains different neurochemical subpopulations with distinct physiological roles. It has been well established that the caudal region of this nucleus is involved in vagal reflexes controlling gastric motility, while the motoneurons with respiration-related activity are located at the rostral-intermediate levels [193].

I.4.1.4 Ambiguous Nucleus

The ambiguous nucleus has a major glossopharyngeal component; it has large neurons. Indeed, it is considered one of the magnocellular nuclei of the respiratory ventrolateral reticular formation, a respiratory center [193].

I.4.1.5 Solitary Tract Nucleus

The solitary tract nucleus consists of neurons of rather small size and is located lateral to the dorsal vagal nucleus. Like the ambiguous nucleus, it is glossopharyngeal, but has small neurons. Viscerosensitive fibers of the glossopharyngeus, coming from the intercarotid and mediastinal baroreceptors are carried along the solitary tract to the solitary tract nucleus. The nucleus has close anatomic relationships with the adjacent vagal nuclei (dorsal vagal nucleus and ambiguous nucleus), with the reticular formation and with the superior centers, particularly the locus coeruleus, and is involved in control of baroreflexogenesis [193].

I.4.1.6 Locus Coeruleus

The locus coeruleus is a complex of catecholaminergic neurons located in the rostral dorsolateral pons, and has been extensively studied in numerous animal species. Projections from this nucleus are responsible for more than half of the noradrenergic connections throughout the brain, including the neocortex, thalamus, amygdala, hippocampus, hypothalamus, cerebellum, medulla oblongata and spinal cord. The locus coeruleus is known to be the major producer of noradrenaline, and subserves several important physiological functions including the sleep-waking cycle and control of the cardiovascular and respiratory systems [141].

I.4.1.7 Hypoglossal Nucleus

The hypoglossal nucleus is the motor nucleus innervating the intrinsic and four of the five extrinsic muscles of the tongue. It is located in the medulla oblongata near the midline, immediately beneath the floor of the inferior recess of the rhomboid fossa. Impairment of deglutition due to hypoplasia and/or neuronal immaturity of the hypoglossal nucleus seems to play a role in SIDS [217].

I.4.2 Spinal Cord

The sympathetic neurons gathered in the lateral horns of levels T1–T5 of the spinal cord send their axons through communicating branches to the ganglia T1–T5 of the sympathetic chain from which the cardiac branches originate. From the first thoracic ganglion the sympathetic trunk extends toward the neck together with the stellate ganglion (cervical inferior, sometimes fused with the first thoracic ganglion), the middle ganglion (small) and the superior cervical ganglion (great), which contribute to the cardiac innervation. The nervous ramifications coming from these ganglionar structures anastomose with those of the vagus nerve [97].

I.4.3 Extrinsic Cardiac Innervation

I.4.3.1 Right Side of the Heart

The nerves of the right side of the human heart, belonging to the right thoracic sympathetic chain, converge in the right stellate ganglion from which originates a thin right stellate cardiac nerve that is directed medially toward the superior vena cava and the aortic sulcus. From the middle cervical ganglion a right dorsolateral cardiac thoracic nerve also originates. The inferior laryngeal recurrent vagus nerve gives off a recurrent cardiac branch and cardiac cranio- and caudovagal nerves [245].

I.4.3.2 Left Side of the Heart

The cardiac innervation of the left portion consists of a prominent sympathetic left stellate ganglion that gives origin to a left stellate cardiac nerve that reaches the left auricula. Most of the left vagal cardiac left branches, in contrast to those of the right, interconnect with the sympathetic branches [245].

All these cardiac nerves, of right and of left, tend to converge in an undefined, varying, but conspicuous extrinsic cardiac plexus (including the intertruncal and/or aorticocoronary plexuses) where there is a rich neuroreceptor paraganglial component. The usual indication of a connection between the aortic and pulmonary glomera is purely conventional.

The first branch of the left coronary artery, sometimes called the intertruncal artery, connects with the system of the paraganglia of the left coronary artery. In the nerve of the extrinsic cardiac plexus there are numerous united cells similar to paraganglial cells (rich in granules containing aminic neurotransmitter) mixed with neurons [241, 245].

I.4.4 Intrinsic Cardiac Innervation

The intrinsic innervation of the heart is represented by a diffused vagal-sympathetic plexus. The plexuses are differentiated into intracardiac, ganglionar, subepicardial, intramyocardial diffused particularly along the coronary ramifications, and terminal to the receptor and afferent structures. The sympathetic neuroreceptors are mostly located in the anterior wall, while the vagal neuroreceptors are in the post-inferior wall. It is almost impossible to distinguish anatomically the sympathetic from the parasympathetic structures, and the afferent from the efferent functions [236].

The vagal and sympathetic nerves, arising or not from the extrinsic cardiac plexus, reach the subepicardium where they form the ganglionar plexus at the level of the sinoatrial inlet of the superior vena cava, around the SAN and along the crista terminalis. Numerous ganglia are gathered around the AV sulcus, but these are rare in the ventricles. The ganglionar sinoatrial plexus is mainly vagal in nature, and seems to decrease from the AV sulcus toward the lower part. From the ganglionar plexus, the so-called "coarse plexus" is branched and divided within the myocardium into a thinner plexus and a terminal or preterminal one. Recently a diagram of the intrinsic cardiac innervation, in which the sympathetic ventricular fibers from the AV sulcus continue into a subepicardial position, from the base toward the apex, becoming intramural and subendocardial, has been proposed. The vagal fibers, instead, cross proximally toward the epicardium and send fibers to the wall and distally to the epicardium near the apex [241].

Regarding the terminal axonal branches, electron microscopy reveals axonal swelling with synaptic vesicles, granular or agranular and rich in neurotransmitters, while the cardiac receptor structures are very difficult to visualize morphologically. Vagal and sympathetic receptors might have different spatial densities in the inferior and anterior ventricular walls [241].

I.4.5 Nervous Structures Regulating Cardiac Activity

In relation to the reflexogenic stimuli of mechano- and chemoreceptor type (variations in cardiac activity in relation to arterial pressure, pO_2 and pCO_2), nervous structures regulating cardiac activity include sympathetic ganglia, carotid cardioinhibitory receptors, and juxtacardiac and mediastinal ganglia and paraganglia.

The sympathetic ganglia comprise the stellate ganglion and the cervicosuperior ganglion.

The carotid cardioinhibitory receptors comprise the carotid body or glomus and the carotid sinus.

The carotid body is a classical chemoreceptor paraganglion, formed principally by cells of neuronal origin whose cytoplasm is rich in argyrophilic granules containing catecholamine neurotransmitter. These cellular elements, gathered in glomeruli (Zellballen), are surrounded by sustentacular cells of schwannian type. The organelles connect with the adventitia of carotid-derived arterioles and with mixed glossopharyngeal nervous plexuses of vagal and less frequently sympathetic origin [97, 181] (Fig. I.7).

The carotid sinus, unlike the carotid body, is a paraganglial organelle. The carotid sinus does not represent a diversified structure, comprising mechanoreceptor glossopharyngeal and in small measure vagal nerve terminations (Krause's club-like), partially anastomosed along the external portion of the middle tunica of the initial tract of the internal carotid artery. The carotid sinus configures an anatomic area inside the arterial tunica media (outer layer), in which many nerve endings (also Krause's club-like) lie. The clear structural difference between the carotid body and the carotid sinus does not correspond to a substantial distinction between, respectively, chemo- and baroreception. In fact, a small paraganglion can sometimes be found in the inside portion of the adventitia of the carotid sinus adjacent to Krause bodies and likewise innervated. Moreover, paraganglial cells are sometimes present in the trunk of the vagus nerve at the level of the carotid bifurcation.

This complex histological structure reflects the difficulty in distinguishing baro- and chemoreflexogenesis in the neuronal glossopharyngeal-vagal circuits of the brainstem [97, 181, 245]. The baroreflexogenic function of the carotid sinus correlates with the chemoreflexogenic function of the inherent glomeruli so forming a unique anatomic complex. Performing a stimulating maneuver, so-called "massage of the carotid sinus" in this region, produces abnormal reflexes provoked not only by the stimulation of the carotid sinus, but also of the local glomerula (carotid body, glomus of the carotid sinus and/or sometimes intravagal paraganglia). Moreover, argyrophilic cells have been observed in the cervical sympathetic ganglia. They are considered interneurons that control the general level of afferent and efferent activity. Experimental evidence suggests that modifications of the cardiac rhythm are due only to the action of the low neuroreceptors rather than to that of the carotid sinus [245] (Fig. I.7).

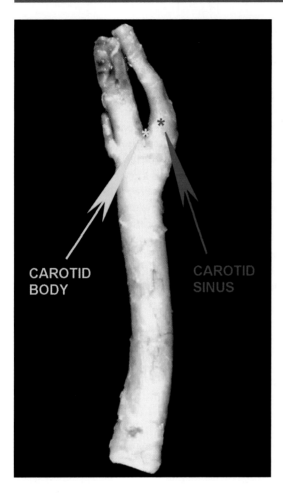

Fig. I.7 The carotid body or glomus is located between the two carotid branches; it is found in the area of the carotid bifurcation, on the internal carotid artery side, close to the "swelling" of the carotid sinus. A little above the bifurcation, the carotid sinus is located just at the root of the internal carotid artery. Modified from a slide contributed by Prof. Simone Gusmão Ramos, University of São Paulo, Brazil

CAROTID
BODY

CAROTID
SINUS

I.4.5.1 Juxtacardiac and Mediastinal Ganglia and Paraganglia

These are situated in the fibroadipose tissue between the ascending aorta, the aortic arch and the bifurcation of the pulmonary artery. They are neuroreceptors, microscopic structures whose fundamental function is to modulate cardiac activity [69]. In the modern literature, different paraganglial structures corresponding to embryonal branchiomeric levels I–IV are distinguished. Beyond the carotid sinuses the mediastinal glomera and the coronary glomus are included. However, the histological picture appears to be more complex: rather than glomera distinguished as "aortic", "pulmonary" and "coronary", minute disseminated receptors are observed, present also in nervous ramifications sometimes with the principal cells mixed with neurons, with no relationship to vascular structures. These ganglial-paraganglial intraneural and extravascular units within the cardiac plexus participate in the regulation, and to the possible disorder, of reflexogenic activity. The juxtacardiac ganglia-paraganglia, as well as the intracardiac receptors, influence the arterial pressure and the cardiac rhythm for vagal and/or sympathetic stimulation [97].

Although there is glomus tissue in a variety of sites throughout the body, the most important are the carotid bodies and the aortic bodies, also known as aortico-pulmonary paraganglia (APP), which are a more diffuse group of small glomera primarily situated in the aortic arch [127]. Little is known about the pathology of the APP. Although they are a critical component of respiratory control, their neuroanatomic complexity has been investigated to only a limited extent in human disease [234, 238]. Histologically they consist of small groups of lobules of glomic tissue separated by a well-vascularized connective tissue with a prolific supply of nerve bundles and ganglion cells [127]. Each lobule contains several distinct cell clusters consisting of central cores of chief (glomus type I) cells surrounded by thin rims of elongated sustentacular (glomus type II) cells [127]. Currently, most investigators consider the chief cells, containing a dense core of neurosecretory granules, to be the chemosensitive element or transducer within the APP with a presumed chemoreceptor function [53]. Only a few investigators have studied the possible role of the APP in pathological processes involving cardiorespiratory disturbances [222].

Materials and Methods

He answered, "While the child was still alive, I fasted and I wept. I thought, "Who knows? The Lord may be gracious to me and let the child live. But now that he is dead, why should I fast? Can I bring him back again? I will go to him, but he will not return to me". (2 Samuel 12:22, 23)

II.1 Clinical and Pathological Information

The procedure for the accurate anatomicoclinical study of each case of infant and perinatal unexplained death includes a review of the clinical history and of the death scene, as well as the anatomicopathological examination. Thus, the guidelines for the investigation include:

- A review of the clinical history
- A detailed description of the death scene (position of the baby in the crib, characteristics and consistency of the pillow and the mattress)
- The anatomo-pathological protocol, to include the gross and histological description of the organs and of the developmental data, and particularly an exhaustive study of the autonomic nervous system, the cardiorespiratory system, the upper digestive pathways, the lungs, and the cardiac conduction system.

For each case of suspected SIDS and unexpected perinatal death referred to our institution, as much clinical information as possible is collected. The review of clinical and epidemiological data, as well as a complete necropsy study, are performed according to the protocol devised by the Institute of Pathology, University of Milan, which is available at: http://users.unimi.it/~pathol/sids_e.html [156, 181, 197].

The value of such a protocol has been recognized internationally. In May 1996 the bill "Post Mortem Regulation on the Sudden Infant Death Syndrome (SIDS) Victims" was presented to the Italian House of Representatives. Since 2000, the Institute of Pathology, University of Milan, has been the coordinating center for a project approved by the Lombardy Region which has the aim of "reduction of the risk of sudden infant death and unexpected fetal death". Since 2002 a Lombardy Region Decree (DGR no. 11693 of 20-06-2002) requires all regional hospitals to perform an autopsy in SIDS infants according to a specific protocol and to refer all the organs to the Institute of Pathology, University of Milan. The form to be used to record the clinical and pathological information in each case is shown in Fig. II.1.

CLINICAL AND PATHOLOGICAL INFORMATION ON THE CASE

Fill in the form and send to Prof. Luigi Matturri, Institute of Pathology, University of Milan, via FAX: +39-02-50320823, or Email: luigi.matturri@unimi.it

CLINICAL AND PATHOLOGICAL FORM FOR THE EVALUATION OF THE RISK FACTORS OF SIDS AND UNEXPECTED PERINATAL DEATH

The present form, in double copy, is integral part of the hospital chart and with it must fully edited by the Hospital personnel. One of the two copies of the card must be send to the data bank of the above-mentioned Institute of Pathology, as devised by the Sanitary Direction.

1. REGISTRY

Referred from (Hospital/Depart.) _____

Ref.# (Hospital Record/Autopsy Record)_____DATE ___/____/_____

LAST NAME:_____ FIRST NAME_____ MIDDLE NAME_____

DATE OF BIRTH:_____/_____/_____ SEX: ☐ M ☐ F____AGE_____

AGE: FETUS: gestational age_____

NEWBORN or INFANT: postocnceptional age___ (gestational age___ +postnatal age)

WEEKS OF GESTATION_____BIRTH WEIGHT (gr.)_____APGAR _____

DATE OF DEATH: _____/_____/_____ TIME_____

PLACE OF BIRTH_____ STATE_____ COUNTRY_____

PERMANENT ADDRESS:

Street Address_____N°_____

Zip/postal Code_____ City_____ State/Province _____

Country_____ Telephone _____

ETHNICITY: ☐ Caucasian   ☐ White Hispanic   ☐ Black   ☐ Oriental

SOCIAL SECURITY#_____

TWIN _____

FEEDING ☐ breast ☐ formula ☐ mixed

When did the formula feeding start? _____

DID THE BABY USE THE PACIFIER? ☐ No   ☐ Yes_____

DATE OF THE LAST VACCINATION_____/_____/ _____

TYPE OF THE LAST VACCINATION _____

DISEASES, ANTENATAL, POSTNATAL OR AT BIRTH_____

SIGNS AND SYMPTOMS:

☐ cold ☐ cough ☐ fever ☐ diarrhea ☐ vomiting ☐ gastro-esophageal reflux
☐ difficult feeding ☐ exanthema ☐ eczema

Fig. II.1 Clinical and pathological information on the case

THERAPIES _____

ELECTROCARDIOGRAMS (ECG) performed on_____at _____

*Attach to this form ECG and copy of the hospital chart including information on the resuscitative maneuvers.

2. FAMILY HISTORY

SIBLINGS

N° _____ SEX _____

AGE _____

HEALTH STATUS _____

MOTHER

LAST NAME_____ FIRST NAME_____ MIDDLE NAME ____

DATE OF BIRTH_____/_____/_____ AGE _____

PLACE OF BIRTH_____ STATE_____ COUNTRY_____

ETHNICITY: ☐ Caucasian ☐ White Hispanic ☐ Black ☐ Oriental

WORK/OCCUPATION_____

LABOR ☐ vaginal delivery ☐ inducted ☐ cesarean delivery

describe: _____

PREGNANCY COURSE _____

PARITY _____

PREVIOUS DELIVERIES_____

N° living births_____N° stillborn_____N° spontaneous abortion _____

N° voluntary abortions_____Dates _____

Date of the last previous delivery_____/_____/_____

CIGARETTE SMOKING before pregnancy: ☐ NO ☐ SI

If NO:

passive smoke exposure at home or at work ☐ NO ☐ SI

describe:_____

If YES:

describe from _____to_____

Cigarettes smoked/day: ☐ 1–5 ☐ 6–10 ☐ 11–20 ☐ more than 20

At what age did you start to smoke?_____

CIGARETTE SMOKING during pregnancy: ☐ NO ☐ SI

If NO:

At what gestational week did you stop smoking?_____

passive smoke exposure at home or at work ☐ NO ☐ SI

Fig. II.1 *(continued)* Clinical and pathological information on the case

describe:_____

If YES:

Cigarettes smoked/day: ☐ 1–5   ☐ 6–10   ☐ 11–20   ☐ more than 20

CIGARETTE SMOKING after pregnancy: ☐ NO   ☐ SI

If NO:

passive smoke exposure at home or at work ☐ NO ☐ SI

specificare:_____

If YES:

describe from _____ to_____

Cigarettes smoked/day: ☐ 1–5   ☐ 6–10   ☐ 11–20   ☐ more than 20

Where do you smoke? ☐ indoor ☐ outdoor: ☐ balcony

COFFEE (n. cups/day) _____

ALCOHOL ☐ No   ☐ Yes _____

DRUGS ☐ No   ☐ Yes_____

MEDICATIONS ☐ No   ☐ Yes _____

CURRENT DISEASES _____

PAST DISEASES_____

DISEASE FAMILIARITY _____

OTHER CASES OF SUDDEN DEATH IN THE FAMILY_____

_____

FATHER

LAST NAME_____ FIRST NAME_____ MIDDLE NAME _____

DATE OF BIRTH_____/_____/_____ AGE _____

PLACE OF BIRTH_____ STATE_____ COUNTRY_____

ETHNICITY: ☐ Caucasian   ☐ White Hispanic   ☐ Black   ☐ Oriental

WORK/OCCUPATION_____

CIGARETTE SMOKING (before, during and after pregnancy) ☐ No   ☐ Yes

From_____to_____

Cigarettes smoked/day: ☐ 1–5   ☐ 6–10   ☐ 11–20   ☐ more than 20

At what age did you start to smoke?_____

COFFEE (n. cups/day) _____

ALCOHOL ☐ No   ☐ Yes _____

DRUGS ☐ No   ☐ Yes _____

MEDICATIONS ☐ No   ☐ Yes _____

CURRENT DISEASES _____

PAST DISEASES_____

DISEASE FAMILIARITY _____

OTHER CASES OF SUDDEN DEATH IN THE FAMILY_____

Fig. II.1 *(continued)* Clinical and pathological information on the case

3. DEATH SCENE

RECOVERY/DEATH PLACE: ☐ HOSPITAL

☐ HOME: ☐ crib/pram   ☐ parents' bed   ☐ stroller, seat, car seat   ☐ in parents' arms

POSITION: ☐ prone   ☐ supine   ☐ on the side

DRESSES _____

When was the last time the baby was seen alive? _____

When was the last meal administered? _____

DATE OF DEATH _____

TIME OF DEATH/WHEN THE BABY WAS FOUND DEAD _____

WHO DID FIND THE BABY DEAD? _____

DATE OF LAST PEDIATRIC VISIT _____/_____/_____

4. AUTOPSY GROSS EXAMINATION

WEIGHT (gr.)_____ CROWN-RUMP LENGTH (cm.)_____

CROWN-HEEL LENGTH (cm.)_____ CRANIAL CIRCUMFERENCE (cm.)_____

THORAX CIRCUMFERENCE (cm.)_____ ABDOMINAL CIRCUMFERENCE (cm.) __

FEET LENGTH (cm.) _____

WEIGHT OF THE ORGANS (gr.):   REMARKS

PLACENTA _____

HEART_____

BRAIN _____

LIVER _____

SPLEEN _____

RIGHT LUNG _____

LEFT LUNG _____

RIGHT KIDNEY_____

LEFT KIDNEY _____

RIGHT ADRENAL GLAND _____

LEFT ADRENAL GLAND _____

THYMUS _____

**Attach copy of autopsy report.

Name and Last Name, Address and Telephone of the pathologist who performed the autopsy_____

_____

Fig. II.1 *(continued)* Clinical and pathological information on the case

II.2 Post-Mortem Regulation on SIDS and Unexpected Fetal Death

The honorable Dr. R. Calderoli, presented to the House of Representatives bill no. 396 of 5 July 2001 "Post mortem regulation on SIDS and unexpected fetal death victims" recently approved by the Senate of the Italian Republic [31, 176].

The problem of SIDS and unexpected fetal death after the 25th week of gestation (unexpected stillbirth) is of great scientific complexity, and the need is therefore clear for anatomicopathological research performed at institutes and departments of pathology, designated as regional referral centers, according to a specific predefined protocol. In every region, the institutes and departments of pathology that are to be referral centers will be designated by special decree. These centers will examine the material and enhance research activity related to this issue. Furthermore, courses should be made available to physicians working in institutes and departments of pathology. Such courses will be aimed at ensuring the uniformity and reproducibility of autopsy techniques and the associated research. An official campaign to raise public awareness of the SIDS issue will be conducted involving the dissemination of appropriate material and the use of the mass media.

Among the industrialized countries, Italy is the only one that does not yet have a national autopsy law relating to SIDS. The Lombardy Region was the first Italian region to approve the "Project for the reduction of the risk of sudden infant death and of fetal unexpected death" (Deliberation of the Regional Government no. 11693 of 20-06-2002). We proposed a remedy for this difficult situation by providing an internationally innovative text in four simple articles at no additional cost to the tax payer. National Law no. 31 of 2/02/06 "Regulations for Diagnostic Post Mortem Investigation in Victims of Sudden Infant Death Syndrome (SIDS) and of Unexpected Fetal Death" designates the Institute of Pathology of the University of Milan as the national referral center (Figs. II.2 and II.3).

II.3 Necropsy Procedure

Infants and fetuses after the 25th week of gestation dying suddenly and unexpectedly are submitted to a complete necropsy examination about 24 hours after death has occurred.

Multiple samples from all organs are fixed in 10% phosphate-buffered formalin, processed and embedded in paraffin, and 5-μm sections are stained with hematoxylin-eosin (H&E). The brain, after fixation, is sectioned in the coronal plane. Multiple samples of the various lobes are fixed and processed, and 5-μm sections are stained with H&E. For the common myocardium, 5-μm sections are stained with H&E and trichromic Heidenhain's (Azan) stain.

In fetuses after the 25th week of gestation considered in our study, the autopsy examination includes a systemic gross and microscopic evaluation of the body, the placental disk, the umbilical cord and membranes. Signs of hypoxic suffering are evaluated using specific criteria based on the presence of subpleural hemorrhagic

SERIE GENERALE

Spediz. abb. post. 45% - art. 2, comma 20/b
Legge 23-12-1996, n. 662 - Filiale di Roma

Anno 147° — Numero **34**

GAZZETTA UFFICIALE

DELLA REPUBBLICA ITALIANA

PARTE PRIMA   **Roma - Venerdì, 10 febbraio 2006**   SI PUBBLICA TUTTI
I GIORNI NON FESTIVI

DIREZIONE E REDAZIONE PRESSO IL MINISTERO DELLA GIUSTIZIA - UFFICIO PUBBLICAZIONE LEGGI E DECRETI - VIA ARENULA 70 - 00100 ROMA
AMMINISTRAZIONE PRESSO L'ISTITUTO POLIGRAFICO E ZECCA DELLO STATO - LIBRERIA DELLO STATO - PIAZZA G. VERDI 10 - 00100 ROMA - CENTRALINO 06 85081

La **Gazzetta Ufficiale**, oltre alla **Serie generale**, pubblica quattro Serie speciali, ciascuna contraddistinta
con autonoma numerazione:

1ª **Serie speciale**: Corte costituzionale (pubblicata il mercoledì)
2ª **Serie speciale**: Comunità europee (pubblicata il lunedì e il giovedì)
3ª **Serie speciale**: Regioni (pubblicata il sabato)
4ª **Serie speciale**: Concorsi ed esami (pubblicata il martedì e il venerdì)

AVVISO AGLI ABBONATI

Si rammenta che la campagna per il rinnovo degli abbonamenti 2006 è terminata il 29 gennaio e
che la sospensione degli invii agli abbonati, che entro tale data non hanno corrisposto i relativi canoni,
avrà effetto nelle prossime settimane.

SOMMARIO

Fig. II.2 Gazzetta Ufficiale of 10 February 2006. In the Table of Contents there is Italian law no. 31 of 2-02-2006. Courtesy of the Istituto Poligrafico e Zecca dello Stato, Rome

LAW N. 31 of 2-02-2006

Regulations for Diagnostic Post Mortem Investigation in Victims of the Sudden Infant Death Syndrome (SIDS) and of Unexpected Fetal Death

Art. 1.

1. Infants that die suddenly within one year of life without any apparent cause, and fetuses that die after the twenty-fifth week of gestation without any apparent cause, must be rapidly submitted, with the consent of both parents, to diagnostic post mortem investigation to be performed in authorized centers, according to the criteria specified in article 2, to which their organs must be sent. Information about the pregnancy, fetal development and delivery and, in the case of sudden infant death syndrome (SIDS), about the environmental and familial situation where the death occurred, must be collected during family interviews, accurately recorded and, to complete the post mortem investigation and for scientific research purposes, assessed by the obstetrician-gynecologist, the neonatologist, the pediatrician involved in the case and the pathologist, in accordance with the international protocols.

2. The post mortem investigation to be set up as in comma 1 are performed according to the diagnostic protocol drawn up by the Institute of Pathological Anatomy, First Chair, University of Milan. To be applicable, the above protocol must be approved by the Ministry of Health.

Art. 2.

Within one hundred eighty days of adoption of the decree as in comma 1, the regions are called upon to individuate in their relative territory, the scientific centers, of University or Hospital appurtenance, that will take on the function of reference centers for the post mortem investigation of infants that die suddenly without any apparent cause within one year of life and of fetuses that die after the twenty-fifth week of gestation, without any apparent cause.

Art. 3.

The results of the post mortem investigation performed as in article 1 will be communicated by the authorized centers to the of the Institute of Pathological Anatomy, First Chair, University of Milan, that will, while fully respecting the norms for the treatment of personal data, set up a national data bank and send the collected data to the competent region, to the general practitioner and pediatricians, and to the relatives of the victim.

Art. 4.

1. The national and regional Health Authorities will be responsible, within the context of the ordinary budget allocation, for:

a) promoting campaigns to ensure awareness and prevention, promulgating correct information about the problems associated with SIDS and unexpected fetal death without any apparent cause;

b) setting up appropriate multidisciplinary research programs carrying out studies of cases from the anamnestic, clinical, laboratory, anatomo-pathological, histological standpoints.

Art. 5.

1. To the charges inherent to the present law, equal to 67.000 Euros annualy, starting in the year 2006, it is provided by correspondent reduction of the enrolled appropriation, for of the triennial budget 2005–2007, within the anticipatory base of current „special Fund" of the Office of the economy and the finances for the 2006, to the purpose partially using the related Ministry budget.

2. The Ministry of the economy and finances is authorized to bring, with own decrees, the required variations of budget.

Fig. II.3 Text of Italian law no. 31 of 2-02-2006 „Regulations for Diagnostic Post Mortem Investigation in Victims of Sudden Infant Death Syndrome (SIDS) and of Unexpected Fetal Death"

petechiae, second-degree depletion of the thymus, marked hepatic erythropoiesis and stress-response pseudofollicular changes of the adrenal gland [47, 171, 274].

In addition to the routine autopsy procedure, our autopsy protocol includes in particular the collection and study of the following structures:

- Cardiac conduction system [161, 210]
- Central, peripheral and autonomic nervous systems
  - Brainstem
    Medulla oblongata
    Pons
    Midbrain [167]
  - Spinal cord
    Cervicothoracic tract [181]
  - Cerebellum [142, 143]
  - Sympathetic ganglia
    Stellate ganglion
    Superior cervical ganglion
  - Carotid bifurcation
    Carotid glomus
    Carotid sinus [236]

- Ganglionic and paraganglionic mediastinal plexuses situated in the fibroadipose tissue between the ascending aorta/aortic arch and the bifurcation of the pulmonary artery [222, 236].

II.4 Cardiac Sampling and Study of the Conduction System

II.4.1 Cardiac Sampling

At the general autopsy, before focusing on the heart, any extracardiac cause of death should be ruled out. The heart is removed in the usual way, but taking the utmost care to sever the great vessels very close to the pericardial reflections. In particular, the superior vena cava should be cut about 2 cm above the pericardial sac to ensure the ability to examine a possibly "high" sinoatrial node (SAN) and of many ganglia of the SAN nerve plexus which extend to the caval funnel adventitia [182, 230] (Fig. II.4).

Determination of the size and weight of the heart should not be omitted, and the values should be compared with normal values for infants of the same length and age [66, 271, 278]. After the presence of gross cardiac malformations has been excluded, the origin of the coronary arteries should be carefully inspected. The heart is systematically examined for pathological changes in the atria, septa, ventricles, pericardium, endocardium and coronary arteries. Samples of the myocardium are stained with H&E and trichromic Heidenhain's (Azan) stain.

Histological examination of the coronary arteries should be carried out according to the following procedure. The major epicardial coronary arteries and branches (left main, anterior descending, left circumflex, right main, posterior descending, right marginal) are excised transversely to their longitudinal axis in segments of approximately 3–4 mm. Each segment is labeled sequentially from either its aortic ostium or its origin from the left main coronary artery. The segments are dehydrated, embedded in paraffin, and sections are stained with H&E and Azan for histological examination, alcian blue (at pH 0.5 and 2.5) for analysis of acid mucopolysaccharides, and Weigert's resorcin-fuchsin stain for identification of elastic fibers. In selected cases, the cells of the walls of the coronary arteries and of the cardiac conduction arteries are immunophenotyped using the immunoperoxidase technique with the following primary antibodies (made from Dako reagents): anti-α-smooth muscle actin to identify smooth muscle cells (SMCs), anti-CD68 to identify monocytes, anti-CD20 and anti-UCHL-1 to identify B- and T-lymphocytes, respectively [172, 175, 177, 183].

II.4.2 Removal of the Cardiac Conduction System Blocks

Histological observations are focused on the cardiac conduction system, which, though fairly constant in layout and structure, shows noteworthy individual variations [154, 238]. Therefore, histological examination of serial sections would be expected to provide the necessary information concerning both topography and pathology of the specialized tissue [181]. The cardiac conduction system is removed

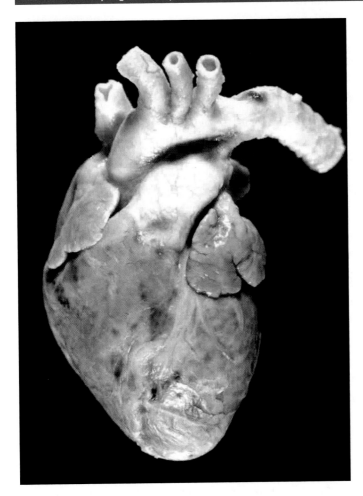

Fig. II.4 At autopsy, the heart should be removed together with a significant length of the great vessels. Determination of the size and weight of the heart should not be omitted, and the values should be compared with normal values for infants of the same length and age. After the presence of gross cardiac malformations have been excluded, the origin of the coronary arteries should be carefully inspected. Slide contributed by Prof. Simone Gusmão Ramos, University of São Paulo, Brazil

in two blocks for paraffin embedding. It is important, in order to "save the pacemaker", to avoid the customary incision of the right heart margin. Instead, the incision should be driven laterally towards the superior vena cava, dividing lengthwise the intercaval bridge. Indeed, using the customary incision, the SAN may be slashed diagonally, together with the crista terminalis. The aorta should always be opened by cutting the mitral aortic valve [230].

According to the sampling technique devised by Rossi [227, 236, 239, 245], two blocks of heart tissue should be removed for paraffin embedding.

Block 1 contains the SAN, its atrial approaches and the crista terminalis, and the SAN ganglionar plexus. The main visual reference for removal is centered upon the sulcus–crista terminalis. Two longitudinal incisions are made parallel to the sulcus–crista line through the atrial wall, with medial extension on the right side to encompass the anterior aspect of the inlet of the superior vena cava. On the left side, one has to section very medially the cava–cava bridge and extend the incision to the superior vena cava wall. Of the two transverse incisions, the superior one is oriented to remove as much as possible of the cava funnel. The inferior incision removes, more or less distally according to the atrial volume, the fan of the pectinate muscles that radiate from the crista terminalis. The procedure for the excision of block 1 is illustrated in Fig. II.5.

Block 2 contains the atrioventricular (AV) system with its atrial approaches. The reference points for the excision are, on the right side, the outlet of the coronary sinus and the pars membranacea septi. Holding the already opened heart so as to expose the interventricular septum against a fairly intense light source, one can clearly see the transparent area of the pars membranacea, which can then be grasped between thumb and index finger. One then proceeds to excise the interventricular septum together with the central fibrous body, the lowermost part of the atrial septum and the adjacent segments of the AV fibrous annuli. The incisions to be made are as follows:

- A longitudinal incision (a) through the posterior part of the septum, across the AV fibrous annulus and up to the superior margin of the coronary sinus ostium.
- A longitudinal incision (b) parallel to a through the superior part of the septum extending to the aortic valvular ring.
- Two incisions perpendicular to a and b to take away the tissue block, with its upper (atrial-aortic) margin about 1.5 cm above the AV ring and its lower (ventricular apex) margin encompassing the base of the medial tricuspid papillary muscle and possibly the moderator band.

The procedure for the excision of block 2 is illustrated in Fig. II.6. After removal, block 2 can be trimmed to regularize its shape by removing the valvular leaflets with the chordae, and the useless tracts of aortic wall and pulmonary conus muscle, well above the pars membranacea.

Some investigators have adopted a technique very similar to the one described above for the excision of tissue block 2, but involving further subdivision of the block into a number of minor fragments which are mounted and sectioned separately. The only advantage of this method is that smaller blocks are presented to special microtomy more suitable for serial sectioning; however, this instrumental advantage is obtained at the cost of occasionally interfering with the fundamental histopathological understanding of the exact extension and layout of damage along the spatially reconstructed AV system and of interfering with the search for mediate accessory AV pathways [263, 264]. It is indeed extremely difficult, if not impossible, to make sections from different fragments coincide with one another in three dimensions, which, in turn, is one of the prerequisites for understanding the arrhythmological pathology of the conduction system.

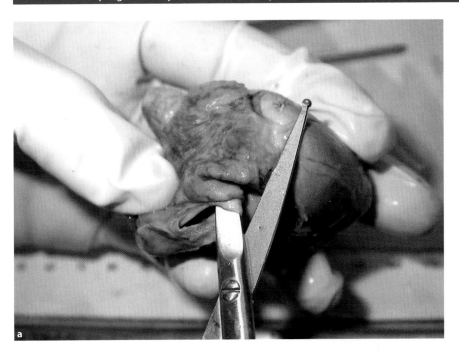

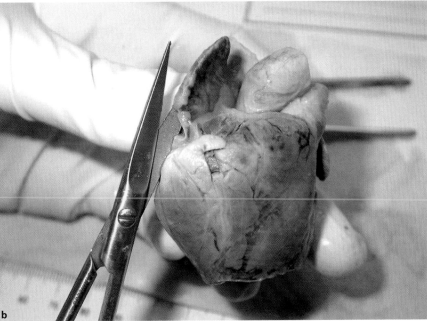

Fig. II.5a–e Excision of block 1 for the study of the cardiac conduction system. **a** The first incision is made from the inferior vena cava along the AV margin. **b** This first excision is extended to the right auricular in the midline. **c–e** *see next page*

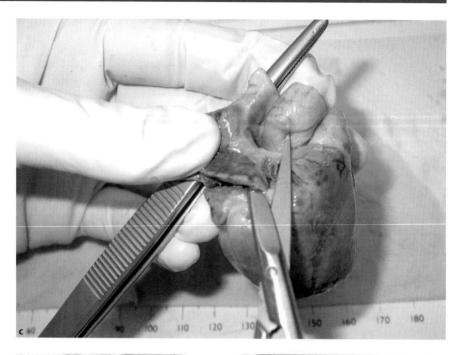

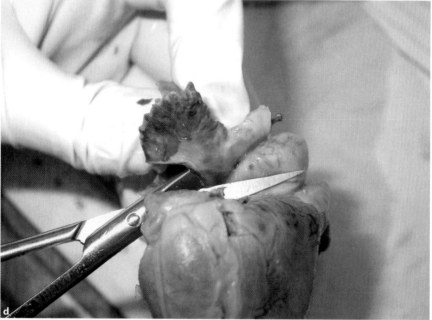

Fig. II.5a–e *(continued)* **c** A second incision is made from the AV line to the superior vena cava. **d** An incision parallel to the crista terminalis is then made. **e** *see next page*

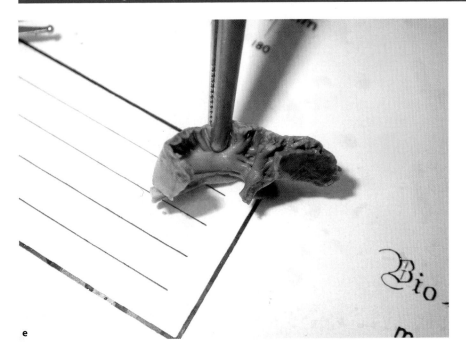

Fig. II.5a–e *(continued)* **e** The block obtained contains the SAN, its atrial approaches, the crista terminalis, and the SAN ganglionar plexus. The main visual reference for the removal is centered upon the sulcus–crista terminalis

Accessory pathways of James and Mahaim type, together with any medial (septoseptal) direct Kent bundles, are included in block 2. Other direct AV accessory bundles of Kent, bridging the AV rings elsewhere, require the examination of both AV annuli in their entirety, with the adjacent muscle, as follows: radial incisions, perpendicular to the plane of the AV ostia, will subdivide the fibrous ring into fragments 1.5–2 cm thick, together with the muscle attached to the ring on both sides; trimming away the free valvular leaflets is suggested.

Our technique for studying the AV junctional tissue and its atrial approaches in the triangle of Koch involves serial sectioning in a plane parallel, i.e. tangential, to the endocardial surface.

II.4.3 Treatment of the Cardiac Conduction Blocks

The two specimens (block 1 containing the SAN and block 2 containing the AV system), excised specifically for the study of the cardiac conduction system are processed manually, with different systems, and further sectioned in series to allow detailed examination, according to the method described by Rossi [230, 236–239, 241].

The two blocks are reduced by removing redundant tissue (papillary muscles and chordae tendinae, etc.) and fixed in 10% phosphate-buffered formalin [2, 43].

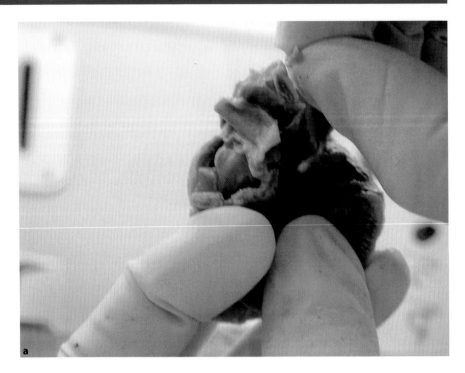

Fig. II.6a–c Excision of block 2 for the study of the cardiac conduction system. **a** Holding the al-ready opened heart so as to expose the interventricular septum against a fairly intense light source, the transparent area of the pars membranacea can be clearly identified. **b, c** *see next page*

Once fixation is complete (3–20 days depending on specimen volume), the forma-lin is removed under running tap water for about 20 minutes. The material is then dehydrated in 95% ethanol for 24 hours followed by four passages in pure dioxan (diethylene dioxide) each for 12 hours. The tissue is then partially impregnated in a mixture of one-third dioxan/two-thirds paraffin (melting point 56–58 °C) and, finally, total impregnated in pure paraffin, both processes being carried out in an oven. Dioxan is the crucial factor in this technique for processing the conduction system since it is both a paraffin solvent and a dehydrator. The more commonly used ethylic dehydration tends to cause the material to become too hard so it breaks upon microtome sectioning [13]. After dehydration, paraffin embedding is carried out using metallic molds for oversized specimens (Fig. II.7).

The blocks must be precisely orientated. For the SAN block, the reference points are the pectinati muscles, that should stand upwards. For the AVN block the aortic semilunar valves should be placed opposite the cut surface. The blocks should be stored in a freezer. The surface paraffin is first removed from each block, and a scal-pel is used to mold all around the block to facilitate sectioning in the microtome and to allow better distension in warm water. The paraffin blocks are better if they are made fairly tall so that they can be caught high in the microtome vice, avoiding the wood or plastic base that tends to become loose.

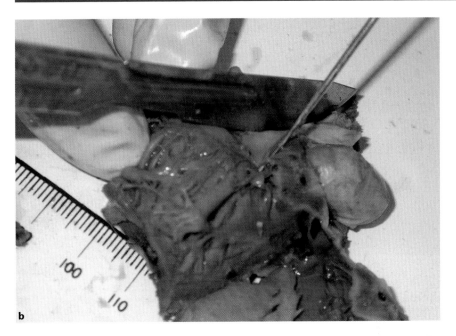

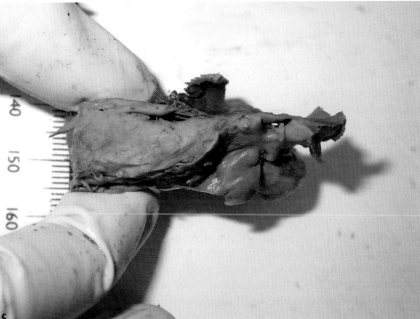

Fig. II.6a–c *(continued)* **b** The interventricular septum is then excised together with the central fibrous body, the lowermost part of the atrial septum and the adjacent segments of the AV fibrous annuli. A longitudinal incision through the posterior part of the septum, across the AV fibrous annulus and up to the superior margin of the coronary sinus ostium is made. **c** Block 2 contains the AV system with its atrial approaches. The reference points of the excision are, on the right side, the outlet of the coronary sinus and the pars membranacea septi.

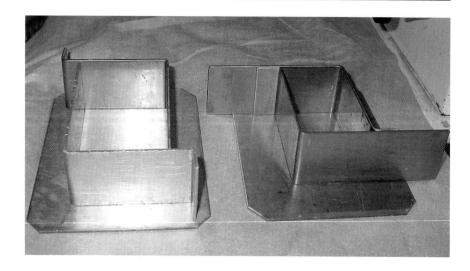

Fig. II.7 The two tissue blocks for the study of the cardiac conduction system after dehydration are embedded in paraffin using metallic molds for oversized specimens

Serial sectioning is an essential part of the investigation of the conduction system, since it allows a further three-dimensional reconstruction of the examined conducting tissue [122, 181]. Depending on the specimen's dimensions, sectioning should be carried out at intervals every 20–40 µm for SAN blocks and every 40–60 µm for AVN blocks, collecting three 8-µm sections at each level. Routine global serial sectioning of the entire specimen would be quite time-consuming, besides the additional work and waste of material [122, 181, 197].

Microscopic evaluation of the slides will enable one to decide whether or not the investigation can be considered ended, in which case the remaining paraffin block can be stored for possible further investigation. The serial sectioning itself can be carried out using a normal manual sledge microtome adapted for tall specimens. The sections obtained can be expanded in warm water at 40–50°C in twin baths, one containing Sta-On tissue section adhesive (Surgipath) for histochemistry, the other without for immunohistochemistry. The sections for immunohistochemistry are collected onto slides pretreated with 3-aminopropyl triethoxysilane (silanized). The slides are previously countersigned and labeled with the number of the case, the paraffin block and the sequence level, and whether silanized or not, and then put in an oven at 37°C overnight. The slides destined for further staining for apoptosis are replaced in the oven at 60°C for 4 hours to enhance the adherence of the section to the glass slide.

For prescreening, it is not necessary to stain specimens from all the levels (for the SAN 70–100, for the AVN 100–130); it may be enough to stain selected specimens from five or six levels alternately with H&E and Azan (acronym for azocarmine/aniline blue stain of Heidenhain).

To obtain good results, before applying the aniline blue, myofibril conducting muscle should be overstained in Azan, developed slowly and blocked with acetic acid, followed finally by the application of phosphotungstic acid as mordant. These Azan solutions are also prepared in the laboratory. Unstained slides are archived for eventual follow-up of the investigations. Various so-called "secondary" stainings are also utilized according to the abnormalities demonstrated.

The histochemical alcian-blue stain, pH 2.5, and periodic acid-Schiff (PAS) stain for acid polysaccharides are used to stain the cartilaginous hypermetaplasia of the heart's central fibrous body from SIDS victims. Alcian blue is also a good stain for circulating and tissue mast cells [13, 147, 220]. Mallory's phosphotungstic acid hematoxylin (PTAH) stain, that we apply with the AFIP (Armed Forces Institute of Pathology) modification with satisfactory results, is similar to Azan and is particularly indicated for morphometric studies and/or for the central nervous system since it stains muscle, elastic fibers, neuroglia, erythrocytes, fibrin and cartilage deep blue, myelin light blue, and cytoplasm, collagen, elastic and reticular fibers, basal membranes and osteoid tissue orange or light-brown [147]. Weigert's method is specific for elastic fibers which stain black or deep brown over a yellow-red background due to Van Gieson's stain for gross connective and muscle tissue. We usually avoid contrast staining with Van Gieson's stain since it fades and disappears in a matter of 10 years. For elastic fibers alone the resorcin-fuchsin method gives quite favorable results [147]. The "slow eosin" method using very dilute eosin (a couple of drops in a beaker of water) gives good results as a differential stain for leukocytes in "critical" preparations, for example in eosinophilic myocarditis. The silanized blank sections can be processed for immunohistochemistry, for example the detection of apoptosis by the TUNEL method for staining fragmented DNA and by PCNA staining, and DAKO S-100 and GFAP for staining neurofibrils [220].

For each heart, the average number of histological sections stained and examined is about 200. The cardiac conduction system can be reconstructed in three dimensions from the series of two-dimensional slides. The same procedure is applicable to material from adults [196, 209, 211].

II.5 Brainstem Sampling

Much emphasis is now laid on the respiratory reflexogenic function of the chemosensitive ventral medullary surface in SIDS [118, 133, 163, 283] and unexpected perinatal loss [167, 171].

The aim of the histological investigation of the human brainstem is to provide basic information on the cardiocirculatory and respiratory central neuronal circuits in order to provide an informed understanding of the inherent histopathological parameters in SIDS and SIUD cases [58, 118, 132, 133, 163, 167, 171].

The brainstem sampling techniques described here, complete and simplified, could allow the general pathologist to cope using a systematic approach with the central neuropathology of SIDS and SIUD or to preserve suitable material for further investigation by specialists, which is much needed to help provide a better understanding of SIDS and sudden unexpected perinatal death.

The examination of the brainstem in SIDS, sudden unexpected perinatal deaths and controls has underlined a remarkable variability, particularly of the arcuate nucleus (ARCn), in both size and neuronal density [58, 118, 120, 133, 163]. Therefore, the complete evaluation of the brainstem and its possible abnormalities requires its examination on serial sections or, in the simplified procedure, the individualization of defined and constant section levels, identifiable through anatomic reference points [120, 174].

In all cases it is important to avoid removing the leptomeninges by tearing, in order to avoid a discontinuity of the ventral medullary surface. The time required for fixation of the brainstem in 10% phosphate-buffered formalin varies from 3–4 days to several days, based on the number of gestational weeks or age of the fetus or infant.

II.5.1 Complete Examination of the Brainstem

In the procedure for complete examination, the brainstem is entirely processed and serially sectioned throughout its entire length. This includes cranially the lower third of the midbrain and caudally the medulla oblongata sectioned some millimeters distally from the lower pole of the inferior olivary nucleus.

In the stillborn and in the newborn the brainstem specimen is processed in its entirety, while in infants, because of its greater size, the brainstem is divided into two parts:

1. The first specimen comprises the medulla oblongata. The upper incision is made some millimeters proximal to the border between the medulla oblongata and the pons; the lower incision is made some millimeters below the lower pole of the olive.
2. The second specimen comprises the pons and the lower third portion of the midbrain.

The brainstem specimen or specimens after fixation is/are dehydrated in ethanol at increasing concentrations and embedded in paraffin with a melting point of 56–58 °C. These passages in ethanol and then in paraffin, to optimize the results, are done manually, varying the times according to the specimen size. The number of serial sections through the entire brainstem varies in relation to the age of the victim. In the fetus, from the 25th week of gestation, the average number of sections is 360, while in the fetus at term and/or in the newborn it is 600. In SIDS victims of 3–4 months and over 6 months of age it is 900 and 1,400, respectively. This procedure allows a detailed evaluation of all the other brainstem nuclei, apart from the ARCn.

In order to apply the appropriate histological staining (H&E, Klüver-Barrera, or trichromic Heidenhain stain) and to perform further histochemical investigations (i.e. Glees-Marsland silver stain for neurons and neurofibrils, Bielschowsky's silver stain for axons and dendrites, Mallory's PTAH stain for glia) and immunohistochemical tests (to study apoptosis, various neuroreceptor structures, the expression of specific genes, etc.), groups of 12 sections are prepared, three of which are used for the histological methods and the other nine saved and stained as deemed necessary for further investigations. Therefore, the number of groups of 12 serial sections varies from 30 in the fetus at the 25th week of gestation (corresponding to 360 sections) to 120 in SIDS victims over 6 months of age (corresponding to 1,400 sections). Therefore, for each case analyzed, and according to the age of the subject, between 90 and 360 sections are stained with H&E, Klüver-Barrera and trichromic Heidenhain stains, and between 270 and 1,080 unstained sections are kept and stained as necessary.

This process represents 4 weeks of work by a histotechnician. Although having the merits of completeness and accuracy, it is not routinely applicable in all histopathological laboratories, for the obvious reason that it requires additional technical personnel [120, 174].

II.5.2 Simplified Examination of the Brainstem

The simplified procedure for the examination of the brainstem of an infant or of the term fetus or newborn requires a much lower number of sections. The cranial, intermediate and caudal portions of the nuclei can be examined, and the technique is applicable in every laboratory. However, this method requires careful and precise sampling.

The brainstem is divided into the following three blocks, as shown in Fig. II.8:

Block I   The cranial block, includes the pontomesencephalic junction.
Block II   The intermediate block, includes the pontobulbar junction.
Block III   The caudal block, corresponding to the submedian area of the inferior olivary eminence, has the obex as a reference point and extends 2–3 mm above and below the obex.

A fourth block (block IV) just below block II can be excised and submitted for genetic analysis.

II.5.3 Treatment of the Brainstem Blocks

The brainstem specimens, after fixation, are dehydrated in ethanol at increasing concentrations and embedded in paraffin with a melting point of 56–58 °C. These passages in ethanol and then in paraffin, to optimize the results, are done manually, varying the times according to the specimen size.

Each block is section transversely at intervals of 30 μm (levels). For each level, twelve 5-μm sections are obtained, three of which are routinely stained for histological examination alternately with H&E, Bielschowsky's and Klüver-Barrera stains, and the other nine are saved and stained as deemed necessary for further investigations. The number of levels and consequently of serial sections through the entire brainstem varies in relation to the age of the victim. In fetuses, from the 30th week of gestation, the average number of sections is 360 (corresponding to 30 groups of 12 serial sections), while in term fetuses and newborns, 600 sections may be ob-

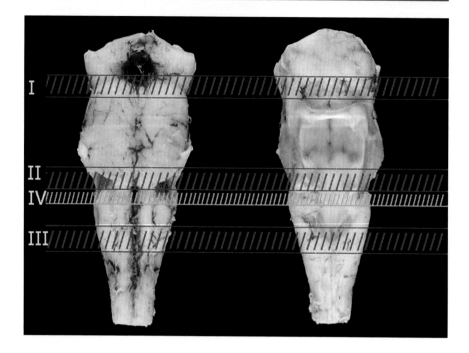

Fig. II.8 Ventral (left) and dorsal (right) surfaces of the brainstem showing the location of the sample blocks I–IV.

tained (30 groups). From infants of 3–4 months and over 6 months of age an average of 900 and 1,400 sections are obtained from 75 and 120 levels, respectively. The important nuclei are demonstrated, namely the ARCn, the hypoglossal nucleus, the dorsal motor vagal nucleus, the solitary tract nucleus, the ambiguous nucleus and the trigeminal tract nucleus, and the ventrolateral reticular formation in the medulla oblongata, together with the locus coeruleus and the parabrachial/Kölliker-Fuse complex in the pons [181].

Two expanding baths are advised, one with Sta-On adhesive and the other without, both at 40–45 °C. Each level requires 12 sections (one for H&E staining, one for Klüver-Barrera staining, six unstained, and four on silanized slides). All are accurately countersigned and put in an oven 37 °C overnight. In the morning the H&E-stained sections are screened in order to decide upon further processing. For morphometry, Klüver-Barrera staining is needed, whereas for apoptosis a prior 4-hour incubation in an oven at 60°C is needed.

H&E staining is advised in all cases. Another method advised is the silver impregnation method of Bielschowsky for axons, dendrites, and nerve cells which are stained black–violet, and in which the "photographic" reduction is obtained by formol, with a final fixing with sodium thiosulfate that renders the silver impregnation permanent [13]. Another method we employ, particularly for the brainstem, is the silver impregnation method of Glees and Marsland for neuronal bodies and neurofibers which are stained black or brown on a bronze-brown lighter background [13]. Mostly in the brainstem the Klüver-Barrera stain is employed for myelin and neurons. It utilizes Luxol fast blue which is derived from tetrabenzotetrazo-porphyrin. The Luxol stain binds with phospholipidic myelin components such as lecithin and sphingomyelin. The Luxol is chromatically contrasted with cresyl violet, which makes it possible to obtain evidence also of cytoplasmic Nissl substance. Mallory's PTAH is also a satisfactory stain for glia, and Azan can be used to show glomic neuroreceptors [13, 147].

II.5.4 Morphometric Analysis

Morphometric analysis is performed with an image analyzer (Image-Pro Plus, Media Cybernetics, Silver Spring, Maryland, USA). For each brainstem nucleus (in particular, the ARCn and the parabrachial/Kölliker-Fuse complex), using serial sections stained with Klüver-Barrera stain, the neuronal cell body areas, neuronal density, transverse section areas and volume are evaluated. Only those neurons with an obvious nucleus and nucleolus are included in the measurements. The profile area of the neuronal bodies is expressed in microns squared, and the transverse sectional area, after delineation of the outer boundaries, in millimeters squared. The neuronal density is evaluated in transverse sections as the number of neurons per millimeter squared. For two-dimensional reconstruction, a computer program developed by Voxblast (Vaytek, Fairfield, Iowa, USA) is used to digitize and align the anatomic boundary tracings in the serial sections [132, 163].

II.6 Study of the Carotid Bifurcation, Ganglia and Paraganglia

II.6.1 Carotid Bifurcation

The carotid bifurcation (right and left) is located at the level of the superior edge of the thyroid cartilage (C4) and is flattened into a Y shape (Fig. I.7). Two receptors at the carotid bifurcation provide feedback to the vasomotor and respiratory centers of the brain: the carotid body and the carotid sinus.

The carotid body or glomus is a highly vascular area located between the two bifurcation carotid branches. It is found in the carotid bifurcation area, on the internal carotid artery side, close to the "swelling" of the carotid sinus (Fig. I.7). The carotid body is a differentiated chemoreceptor paraganglion, formed principally by cells of neuronal origin whose cytoplasm is rich in argyrophilic granules of catecholamine neurotransmitter. These cellular elements, gathered in glomeruli ("zellballen") are surrounded by sustentacular cells of schwannian type. The organelle is in strict connection with the adventitia of arterioles of carotid derivation and with mixed glossopharyngeal nervous plexuses which are vagal and less frequently sympathetic [97,

181]. The carotid body functions as a chemoreceptor sensitive to blood oxygen concentration (pO$_2$) and, to lesser extent, blood pH and the partial pressure of carbon dioxide (pCO$_2$) [174].

The carotid sinus is located a little above the bifurcation, just at the root of the internal carotid artery. The carotid sinus delineates an anatomic area inside the arterial media (outer layer), wherein many nerve endings (also Krause's club-like) lie. However, even in this area (well outside the carotid body) some small glomera can be recognized microscopically. For this reason it is better not to draw too clear-cut topographic boundaries between chemoreceptors (paraganglia) and baro- or mechanoreceptors (intercarotid nerve endings). The carotid sinus is a fusiform dilatation that functions as a baroreceptor to monitor blood pressure [174].

The carotid bifurcations are separately embedded in paraffin and serially sectioned.

II.6.2 Mediastinal Ganglionic and Paraganglionated Plexuses

The soft adipose fibrous (fascial) tissue between the aortic and pulmonary trunk (intertruncal plexuses), and between the aortic arch and the pulmonary hili, is removed. Sectioning the fragments in series reveals the cardiac plexus ganglia and paraganglia. The left coronary artery neuroglomic plexus should be sought at the root of the artery; sometimes the tiny intertruncal artery can be glimpsed (almost never quoted in the textbooks). The plexuses are embedded well, compressing the fatty tissue on the cutting surface. The structures to be examined are invisible to the naked eye, so the maximal surface needs to be examined in each section.

II.6.3 Cervical Sympathetic Ganglia

In term fetuses and in infants, while taking out an "abundant" intercarotid block of tissue, the superior cervical ganglion can be found; the middle cervical ganglion is inconstant, while the stellate ganglion (inferior cervical often fused with the first thoracic) can be found close to the branching of the subclavian and vertebral arteries. The ganglia can be embedded complete, or can be divided longitudinally, but further examined together.

The carotid bifurcation, mediastinal and aorticopulmonary ganglia and paraganglia, adequately labeled, are fixed in buffered formalin. In infants, we recommend that the excision of these structures be carried out on already fixed material. The material should be washed in tap water immediately after fixation. The dehydration of these tissues is different from that used for the conduction system study [2]. The ablated fragments have a soft consistency and it is better to use a dehydration that will harden up the specimens. We use ethylic alcohol at increasing concentrations (70%, 95% in two changes, 100% in two changes) and then xylol in two changes, which is followed by embedding in two changes of pure paraffin at a melting point of 56–58 °C in the oven. The changes are best carried out manually because of the different times required depending on the specimen dimensions. The embedded material is serially sectioned.

II.7 Lung: Evaluation of the Stage of Development

In each SIUD case and unexpected neonatal death the stage of pulmonary development is evaluated on the basis of a macroscopic criterion used at autopsy, namely the ratio between lung weight and body weight (LW/BW), and according to microscopic criteria, that is, the presence of cartilaginous bronchi up to the distal peripheral level and the radial alveolar count (RAC). Determination of the RAC involves examining at least ten fields for each case (with a ×40 lens) in order to estimate the number of alveoli transected by a perpendicular line drawn from the center of the most peripheral bronchiole (recognized by being incompletely covered by epithelium) to the pleura or the nearest interlobular septum. For this examination, we use samples of fetal lung sectioned parallel to the frontal plane and passing through the hilus.

The normal reference values for the last 3 months of gestation are >0.022 for LW/BW and the range 2.2–4.4 for RAC [10, 171].

II.8 Immunohistochemistry and Other Techniques

In selected cases, immunohistochemistry studies are performed on sections of the cardiac conduction system, brainstem, and coronary arteries.

II.8.1 Apoptosis

The sections are deparaffinized and incubated with 20 µg/ml proteinase K (Sigma, St. Louis, MO, USA). After blocking the endogenous peroxidase with 3% H_2O_2, deoxynucleotidyl transferase (TdT 0.3 U/ml) is used to add digoxigenin-conjugated deoxyuridine (dUTP 0.01 mM/ml) to the ends of DNA fragments. The signal of TdT-mediated dUTP nick end labeling (TUNEL) is then detected by an anti-digoxigenin antibody conjugated with peroxidase (ApopTag peroxidase in situ apoptosis detection kit; Oncor, Gaithersburg, MD, USA). Apoptotic nuclei are identified by the presence of dark-brown staining. Counterstaining is performed by immersing the slides in methyl green for 10 minutes. The apoptotic index (AI) is defined as the number of apoptotic cells divided by the total number of cells counted, expressed as a percentage, as previously described [162, 203].

II.8.2 Proliferating Cell Nuclear Antigen (PCNA)

Paraffin sections are cut and mounted on glass slides and air-dried at room temperature overnight. Sections are deparaffinized and immersed in TRIS-HCl buffered saline solution (TBS, pH 7.6). After blocking the endogenous peroxidase with 3% H_2O_2, the sections are immunostained with the monoclonal PC10 antibody (dilution 1:200) using the avidin biotin (ABC) complex method with overnight incubation. Diaminobenzidine is used as a chromogen, and a light hematoxylin counterstain is used. Biotinylated rabbit anti-mouse IgM is used as a secondary antibody (Vectastain ABC kit; Vector Laboratories, Burlingame, CA, USA). All incubations are carried out in a humidified chamber at room temperature, and, after each incubation, the slides are extensively washed with three changes of TBS. Inflamed palatine tonsils are used as positive controls for PCNA. The PCNA labeling index (PCNA-LI) is defined as the number of cells with strong unequivocal nuclear staining, divided by the total number of cells counted, expressed as a percentage, as previously described [130, 202].

II.8.3 c-Fos

Sections are deparaffinized in xylene and rehydrated. Endogenous peroxidase is blocked by incubation with 3% hydrogen peroxide for 5 minutes. After washing in phosphate-buffered saline (PBS), the sections are incubated with 10% normal goat serum and then with 1:100 diluted polyclonal anti-c-fos antibody (SC-52P, Santa Cruz Biotechnology, CA, USA) at room temperature for 1 hour. After washing in PBS for 5 minutes, the sections are incubated with biotinylated goat anti-rabbit IgG antibody supplied in the kit for 30 minutes, incubated with streptavidin-peroxidase for 30 minutes, stained with 3,3´-diaminobenzidine tetrahydrochloride (DAB, Sigma) solution (30 mg DAB and 0.5 ml 0.3% hydrogen peroxide in 100 ml 0.05 M TRIS-HCl, pH 7.6) and counterstained with cresyl violet. In order to confirm the specificity of c-fos immunostaining, sections from every case are also treated with a blocking peptide (final concentration 10 µg/ml, SC-52P; Santa Cruz Biotechnology), coincubated with the anti-c-fos antibody and then treated in the same way.

In selected cases, the nuclei of the medulla oblongata (in particular the hypoglossal, dorsal motor vagal, solitary tract, ambiguous, arcuate and inferior olivary nuclei) are examined for c-fos immunoreactivity. Neurons are defined as positive when a clear brown staining is present, stronger than in the surrounding interstitium. To evaluate the distribution of c-fos immunostaining in the nuclei of the medulla oblongata, a qualitative rating system is used at each level examined (rostral, intermediate and caudal, respectively), ranging from − to +++. Briefly, the scoring system for each brainstem nucleus is: −, no c-fos-positive cells; +, a few dark c-fos-positive cells (<10%); ++, a moderate number of c-fos-positive cells ranging from 10% to 50%; and +++, a high number of c-fos-positive cells (>50%) [131].

II.8.4 Fluorescence In Situ Hybridization (FISH)

In selected cases, coronary and carotid arteries are studied using FISH.

We use an α-satellite DNA probe specific for the centromeric region of chromosome 7, labeled with biotin (Oncor). The centromeric probe is prepared by mixing 1.5 µl of the probe with 30 µl of Hybrisol VI (Oncor). The probe is applied to the prepared air-dried slides (15 µl) and coverslipped. Both probes and target DNAs are denatured by placing the slides on a hot-plate at 67±2 °C for 5 minutes followed by incubation overnight in a prewarmed humidified chamber at 37 °C. The hybridized signals are detected using a commercial kit (FITC avidin detection kit, Oncor). An antifade solution containing propidium iodide 2.5 µg/ml is used for counterstaining. A Leitz Orthoplan with a Ploemopak incident-light fluorescence microscope, equipped with ultraviolet excitation filter sets, is used for scoring. Only interphase cell nuclei with intact morphology are scored. The number of hybridization spots in each cell is determined [139].

II.8.5 α-Actin Immunohistochemistry

In coronary arteries, to identify neointimal cells as smooth muscle cells (SMCs), additional immunohistochemical staining with the avidin-biotin method is performed with a monoclonal antibody against α-actin (Renner, Dannstadt, Germany) [175].

II.9 Cases Analyzed

From 1987 to 2003, at the Institute of Pathology, University of Milan, many cases of sudden infant and fetal death have been analyzed, since the Institute is the Reference Center for the Lombardy Region for SIDS and late unexplained fetal death (DGR no. 11693 of 20-6-2002). Ethical consent is not required for our study as the Institute of Pathology is the National Referral Center for the Study of Sudden Unexpected and Unexplained Infant and Perinatal Death, according to Italian law no. 31 of 2-02-2006 "Regulations for Diagnostic Post Mortem Investigation in Victims of Sudden Infant Death Syndrome (SIDS) and Unexpected Fetal Death".

From among an even larger number of cases, a total of 120 SIDS victims, 37 infant controls and 60 late fetal stillbirths were selected for this work, after exclusion of violent causes.

II.9.1 SIDS Cases

The cases were classified as SIDS victims when death was sudden, completely unexpected, and unexplained after a thorough case investigation, including a complete autopsy, examination of the death scene, and review of the clinical history [280]. SIDS victims eligible for this study were those who died suddenly and unexpectedly and whose autopsy findings did not have any other explanation than SIDS [273]. The SIDS group considered in this study comprised 81 males (67.5%) and 39 females (32.5%) (Fig. II.9), ranging in age from 3 to 416 days (mean±SEM 91.90±9.55 days).

For the study of the cardiac conduction system, since SIDS occurs most commonly between 2 and 4 months of age [80, 86, 185] and postnatal morphogenesis of the cardiac conduction system is age-related [87, 88, 91], we divided the SIDS infants into three subgroups: (1) from 3 to 60 days, (2) from 61 to 120 days, and (3) from 121 to 365 days.

For each case of SIDS submitted to our institute, our purposes were to verify the diagnosis of SIDS, whether there were any common pathological findings among the SIDS victims, and to suggest areas for further research.

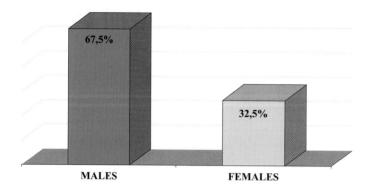

Fig. II.9 The SIDS cases were 81 males (67.5%) and 39 females (32.5%).

II.9.2 "Gray Zone" SIDS Cases

"Gray zone" or borderline SIDS cases are defined as those infants in whom it is difficult to establish if a specific microscopic finding is sufficiently severe to have caused
the death [273].

In some of our cases that had been considered SIDS after an accurate autopsy
performed at other institutions, further investigations of the brainstem in serial sections at our institute revealed important anatomicopathological findings that cast
doubt on the classification as SIDS [159, 160, 213, 214].

II.9.3 SIUD Cases

A case is classified as SIUD when after the 25th week of gestation the fetus dies
suddenly and without explanation before complete expulsion or removal from the
mother [42, 115, 171].

In all of our stillborn fetuses, the brainstem and the cardiac conduction system
were studied in serial sections. Among the SIUD victims, the coronary arteries
were studied in 22, and 13 were male and 9 were female ranging in age from 32 to
40 weeks of gestation [172].

II.9.4 Explained Death Cases

The control group was represented by term fetuses, newborns and infants who
had died of various documented causes, including in particular accidental cranial trauma, generalized sepsis, necrotizing enterocolitis, hypertrophic cardiomyo-
pathies, etc.

In some cases submitted to our institute with a clinical and even post-mortem
diagnosis of SIDS, the study of the cardiac conduction system and brainstem in serial sections disclosed a precise cause of death [204].

For the study of the cardiac conduction system, the control infants, in a similar manner to the SIDS victims, were divided into three subgroups, according to age: (1) from 3 to 60 days, (2) from 61 to 120 days, and (2) from 121 to 365 days.

II.10 Statistical Analysis

Quantitative data were expressed as means±SEM. The data were analyzed using SPSS software. The significances of differences between parameters of the two fetus groups (SIUD and stillborn controls) and two infant groups (SIDS and infant controls) were evaluated using Student's t test for uncoupled data, and the chi-squared test. The level of significance chosen was p<0.05, two-tailed.

Results

Death has climbed in through our windows and has entered our fortresses; it has cut off the children from the streets and the young men from the public squares. (Jeremiah 9:21)

III.1 Epidemiological Results

Regarding the SIDS infants, the risk factors for SIDS proposed by Guntheroth and Spiers [73, 74, 77] were considered in this study:

- Infant factors: sex [188], age [80, 86], prematurity [80, 149], low birth weight [23], family association with SIDS, season [123], sleep prone position [75] (Table I.1);
- Maternal factors: cigarette smoking [122, 133, 257], drugs, alcohol age, marital status, socioeconomic status [9] (Table I.1).

Regarding SIUD, the epidemiology is still largely unknown and was an object of the study. Advances in maternal and fetal care have produced a significant reduction in perinatal mortality, but have not changed the prevalence of SIUD [171, 174].

The total cases investigated were: 120 SIDS victims, 37 infant controls, and 60 late fetal stillborns.

III.1.1 Age

The age distribution of the SIDS infants is shown in Fig. III.1. In particular, 21% of deaths occurred in the 2nd month, 22% in the 3rd, 13% in the 4th, and 10% in the 5th.

III.1.2 Sex

The SIDS group consisted of 81 males (67.5%) and 39 females (32.5%), ranging in age from 3 to 416 days (mean±SEM 91.90±9.55 days). The remarkable prevalence of the male sex is self evident (Fig. II.9).

SIDS CASES

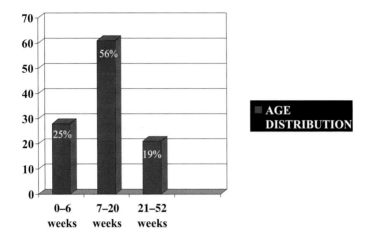

Fig. III.1 Age distribution of SIDS victims

III.1.3 Season

SIDS occurred more frequently in winter and fall, as shown in Fig. III.2. The distribution of SIDS according to the month was: 16% in January, 10% in February, 8% in March, 4% in April, 12% in May, 5% in June, 5% in July, 1% in August, 4% in September, 9% in October, 12% in November, and 14% in December. The peak was in January and the lowest in August.

III.1.4 Time

Most of the SIDS infants died between 10.00 p.m. and 8.00 a.m. (62%); 47% died between 8.00 a.m. and 2.00 p.m., 7% between 2.00 p.m. and 6.00 p.m., and 9% between 6.00 p.m. and 10.00 p.m.

III.1.5 Death Scene: Place of Death

Most of the SIDS infants were found dead in the crib or pram (87%); 3% were in a stroller, seat or car seat, 4% at kindergarten, 4% in hospital, 4% in the parents' bed, and 2% in the parents' arms (Fig. III.3).

III.1.6 Death Scene: Position in the Crib

Most of the SIDS infants died in a prone position (52%); 46% were in a supine position and 2% were lying on their side (Fig. III.4).

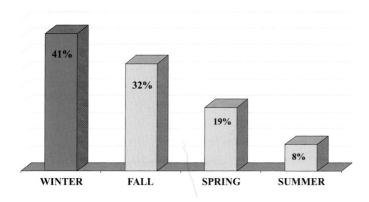

Fig. III.2 SIDS occurred more frequently in winter and fall

SIDS CASES

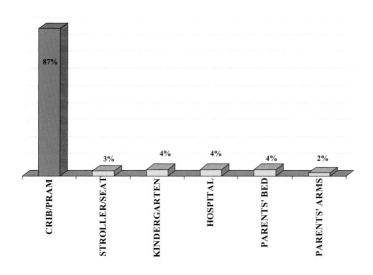

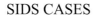

Fig. III.3 SIDS distribution according to the place of death

III.1.7 Feeding

Of the SIDS infants, 36% were breast-fed, 40% were formula-fed, and in 24% feeding was mixed (about 50% formula and 50% human milk) (Fig. III.5).

SIDS CASES

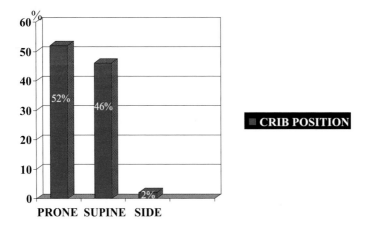

Fig. III.4 SIDS distribution according to position in the crib

SIDS CASES

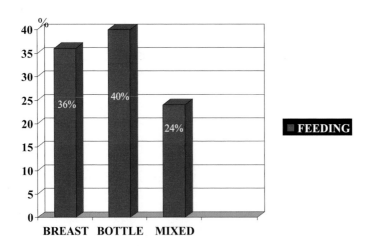

Fig. III.5 Feeding: 36% of SIDS infants were breast-fed, 40% were formula-fed, and in 24% feeding was mixed (about 50% formula and 50% human milk)

III.1.8 Cigarette Smoke Exposure

In about 55% of both SIDS and SIUD victims, at least one parent was a smoker and, generally, smoked more than five cigarettes a day. In the mothers, the smoking habit had started before pregnancy. Cigarette smoking was significantly associated with structural alterations in the arcuate nucleus (ARCn) [133]. These alterations included bilateral hypoplasia, monolateral hypoplasia, partial hypoplasia, delayed neuronal maturation, decreased neuronal density. In about one-third of SIDS cases, formula feeding was combined with cigarette smoking by one or both parents [172, 175].

III.2 Cardiac Conduction Findings

Crib death infants do not show any abnormality of the ordinary myocardium, while the core of the heart, where the cardiac rhythm arises and spreads, shows some abnormalities [210].

The cardiac conduction systems of 100 SIDS victims and 24 victims of explainable death were studied. No significant differences were found between the SIDS and the explainable death groups and subgroups with regard to mean age of the infants (Student's t test), nor were there significant differences between sexes ($\chi 2$ test). The demographic data of the infants and cardiac conduction histological findings for the two groups are presented in Fig. III.6.

More than one cardiac conduction change was present in the same infant, but no unusual combined cardiac anomalies [64] were observed.

III.2.1 Resorptive Degeneration

We observed areas of resorptive degeneration in 97% of the SIDS infants and in 75% of the controls (Fig. III.6). Statistical analysis showed a significant difference between the two groups ($p<0.05$). In the resorptive degeneration areas we observed clusters of young fibroblasts depositing collagen caught in the central fibrous body, sometimes isolated from the overdeveloped specialized structures, and sometimes adjacent to them [87, 198]. In these areas there was no associated inflammation nor any massive necrosis or hemorrhage. Macrophages were sometimes present adjacent to the small foci of degeneration, acting eventually as scavenger cells [95, 161, 210] (Fig. III.7).

III.2.2 Atrioventricular Node and Bundle of His Dispersion/Septation

Dispersion or septation of the bundle of His [11, 238], characterized by fragmentation of the main bundle within the central fibrous body [161, 210, 264], was observed in 33% of SIDS infants and in 17% of the controls, without a statistically significant difference ($p>0.05$) (Fig. III.6).

Atrioventricular node (AVN) dispersion or septation [161, 199, 210] was present in 7% of SIDS infants, but was not detected in the controls.

CARDIAC CONDUCTION SYSTEM

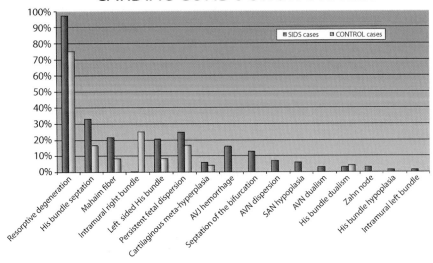

Fig. III.6 Cardiac conduction system findings in SIDS infants and controls

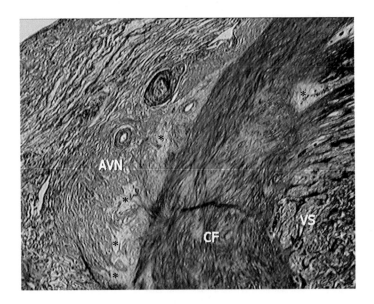

Fig. III.7 Cardiac conduction system. Areas of resorptive degeneration (asterisks), located at the periphery of the atrioventricular node (AVN) and embedded in the central fibrous body (CF) (VS interventricular septum; trichromic Heidenhain, ×25)

III.2.3 Persistent Fetal Dispersion

Islands of conduction tissue in the central fibrous body, designated as persistent fetal dispersion [103, 116, 264], were found in 25% of SIDS infants and in 17% of controls. In such cases we observed islands of conduction tissue separated from the AVN and bundle of His, dispersed in the central fibrous body, resembling the normal fetal pattern [91, 103, 210, 264]. There was no statistically significant difference between the two groups (p>0.05) (Fig. III.8).

III.2.4 Accessory Pathways

Mahaim fibers, specialized connections between the AV junction and the upper ventricular septum [161, 181, 236, 238], were detected in 23% of SIDS infants and in 8% of controls. There was no statistically significant difference between the two groups (p>0.05) (Figs. III.6 and III.9).

Kent fibers, defined as direct accessory pathways outside the AV junction [178], are the morphological substrate for the Wolff-Parkinson-White (WPW) syndrome [36, 136, 181, 193]. They were detected in two SIDS infants (2%), but were not detected in the controls.

James fibers, defined as atriohissian accessory pathways connecting the right atrium directly with the bundle of His [193], were observed in two SIDS infants (2%), but were not detected in the controls.

III.2.5 Cartilaginous Metahyperplasia/Hypermetaplasia

Cartilaginous metahyperplasia of the central fibrous body [210, 238] was present in 6% of SIDS infants and in 4% of controls. There was no statistically significant difference between the two groups (p>0.05) (Figs. III.6 and III.10).

III.2.6 Hemorrhage of the Cardiac Conduction System

Hemorrhage of the AV junction [5] was present only in SIDS infants (16%). We considered hemorrhage to be present only when red blood cells were seen in the intercellular spaces. In some SIDS infants the red cells were widely dispersed over an area of specialized myocardium, and in others discrete clumps of red cells were present enclosing several working as well as specialized myocardial fibers.

III.2.7 Intramural Right Bundle Branch

Intramural right bundle branch was present, respectively, in 20% of SIDS infants and in 25% of the controls. There was no statistically significant difference between the two groups (p>0.05) (Figs. III.6 and III.11).

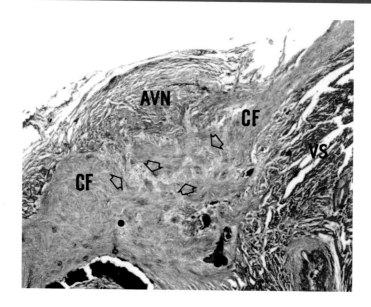

Fig. III.8 SIDS case. Persistent fetal dispersion. Arrows point to islands of junctional tissue separated from the atrioventricular node (AVN), dispersed in the central fibrous body (CF), some of which are undergoing resorptive degeneration (•) (VS interventricular septum; trichromic Heidenhain, ×25)

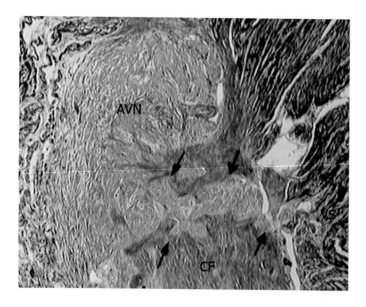

Fig. III.9 Nodoventricular accessory Mahaim fibers (arrows) likely residual from defective resorptive degeneration, bridging the atrioventricular node (AVN) and the ventricular septum (VS) through the central fibrous body (CF) (trichromic Heidenhain, ×25)

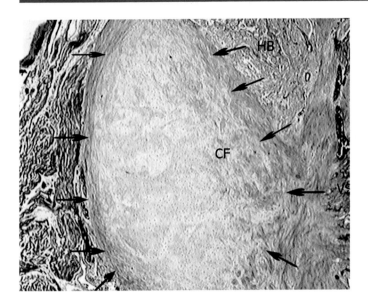

Fig. III.10 Cartilaginous hypermetaplasia (CM) within the central fibrous body (CF, arrows) (HB bundle of His, VS interventricular septum; trichromic Heidenhain, ×25)

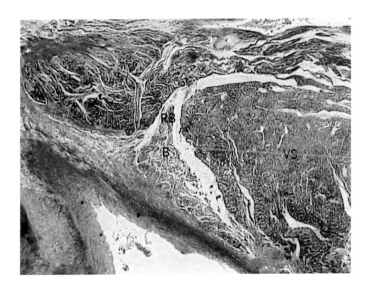

Fig. III.11 Left sided bifurcation (B) and intramural right bundle branch (RB) (VS interventricular septum; trichromic Heidenhain, ×25)

III.2.8 Left-Sided Bundle of His

A left-sided bundle of His [22, 154] was present in 20.29% of SIDS infants and in 8.3% of infants with explainable death. There was no statistically significant difference between the two groups (p>0.05). In one infant the bundle of His was left-sided and intramural (Figs. III.6 and III.12).

III.2.9 Intramural Left Bundle Branch

Intramural left bundle [229] was observed in 2% of SIDS infants, and in none of the controls (Fig. III.6).

III.2.10 Septation of the Bifurcation

Septation of the bifurcation, known also as anomalous bifurcation [161, 238], characterized by interposition of fibrous tissue of the central fibrous body, was detected in 13% of SIDS infants, and in none of the controls (Fig. III.13).

III.2.11 Hypoplasia of the Cardiac Conduction System

Hypoplasia of the sinoatrial node (SAN) [22, 238] was present in 6% of SIDS infants, but was not present in infants with explainable death (Fig. III.6).

Hypoplasia of the bundle of His was present in 5% of SIDS infants but in none of the controls (Fig. III.6).

III.2.12 Atrioventricular Node/Bundle of His Dualism

Dualism of the AVN [201, 241] was present in 3% of those SIDS infants who died between 3 and 120 days of life (Fig. III.14), but in none of those with explainable death. Dualism of the bundle of His was present in 3% of SIDS infants and in 4% of the controls. In these cases the AVN and/or the bundle of His appeared stratified into two portions by the interposition of a fibrous diaphragm [161, 210] (Fig. III.6).

III.2.13 Zahn Node

A Zahn node, also known as a coronary sinus node [158, 227], was present in 3% of the SIDS infants but in none of the controls. In these cases, close to the major axis of the AVN, a formation composed of myocytes of small size and lengthened or stellate in shape arranged with a muscular network was observed, morphologically definable as a small AVN. A typical feature of a Zahn node is a posterosuperior prolongation with a pseudohissian fascicle (Fig. III.6).

III.2.14 Fibromuscular Hyperplasia of the Conduction System Arteries

In 21% of SIDS infants a thickening of the SAN and/or AVN artery was observed. This thickening consisted of fibromuscolar hyperplasia of the cardiac conduction

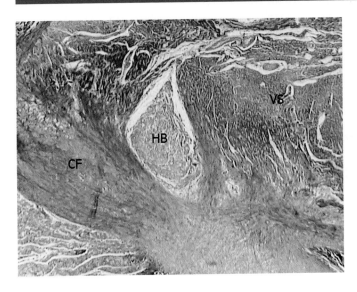

Fig. III.12 Intramural left-sided bundle of His (HB) penetrating the interventricular septum (VS) (CF central fibrous body; trichromic Heidenhain, ×25)

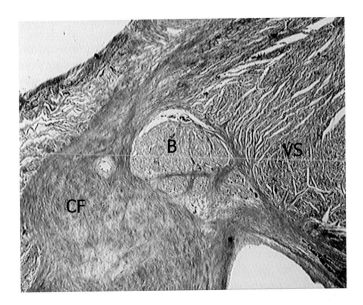

Fig. III.13 Anomalous bifurcation (B) characterized by interposition of fibrous tissue of the central fibrous body (CF) (VS interventricular septum; trichromic Heidenhain, ×25)

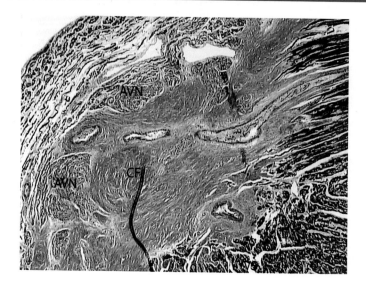

Fig. III.14 The atrioventricular node (AVN) is subdivided into two portions by interposition of fibrous tissue of the central fibrous body (CF) (VS interventricular septum; trichromic Heidenhain, ×25)

system arteries [210] attributable to an initial preatherosclerotic lesion. A significant correlation between these lesions and parental cigarette smoking was found (p<0.05) [177].

The initial preatherosclerotic lesions related to cigarette smoking were detectable in the first few months of life. The atherogenic effects of formula feeding were detectable after the 4th month of life, and worsened if the formula feeding was prolonged [175, 177].

The more diffuse initial preatherosclerotic lesions were seen in formula-fed babies with smoker parents, possibly due to the combined effect of the two pathogenic noxae. These lesions were marked by significant fragmentation of the elastic fiber system and deposits of amorphous material, mainly lipids, even in the innermost portion of the media [175, 177] (Fig. III.15).

III.2.15 Apoptosis Expression in the Conducting Tissue

In this study, the apoptotic indices (AI) in the cardiac conduction system of SIDS infants (range 0.80–4.50; mean±SEM 2.45±0.44) and in controls (range 2.79–3.00; mean±SEM 2.89±0.05) showed no statistically significant differences (p>0.05; Student's t test), while in the resorptive degeneration areas the AI was found to be higher in the controls than in the SIDS infants (p<0.05; Student's t test). The SAN in both groups showed AIs similar to those in the common myocardium. In almost all cases, TUNEL labeling was detected in the peripheral region of the AVN, close to

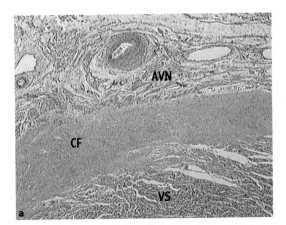

Fig. III.15a,b Myointimal thickness of the atrioventricular node artery in a 4-month-old child who died suddenly and unexpectedly. Not the increased amount of mucoid ground substance in the subendothelial connective tissue (AVN atrioventricular node, CF central fibrous body, VS interventricular septum; H&E, a ×25, b ×100)

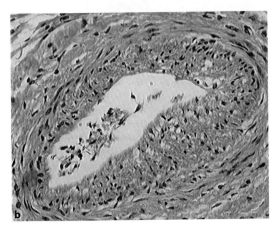

the atrial myocardium (Fig. III.16). The AI were higher in the AVN, the bundle of His and in the initial tract of the bundle branches than in the common myocardium (p<0.05; Student's t test) [162, 207].

III.2.16 PCNA Expression in the Conducting Tissue

Positive PCNA immunoreactivity was not found either in the SIDS infants or in the controls, nor in the conducting system or the common myocardium.

III.2.17 ECG Findings

One or more ECG recordings were available in 15% of the SIDS infants. The ECGs recorded at the time of arrival at hospital when resuscitative efforts were attempted showed that five infants had ventricular fibrillation, and two had supraventricular tachycardia. In six infants the ECGs, recorded mostly soon after birth because of

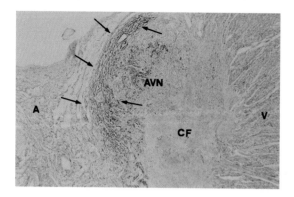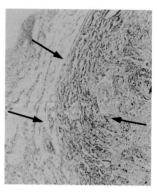

Fig. III.16a,b Apoptotic cells (stained brown, arrows) located at the periphery of the atrioventricular node (AVN) close to the atrial myocardium (A) (VS ventricular septum, CF central fibrous body; TUNEL, a ×20, b ×100)

prematurity problems, were unremarkable; in two patients the ECGs showed long QT syndrome [161].

In a 3-month-old boy dying of SIDS, who was submitted to external cardiac massage for a total of 90 minutes in two successive bouts, the heart resumed sporadic beating 16 hours from the start of resuscitation attempts (aided by sporadic emergency maneuvers) for a few hours, with ECG findings of right branch block and downsloping of the ST segment, but no clear-cut sign of ischemia. The baby remained unconscious and was pronounced dead 26 hours after hospitalization. At the post-mortem examination, in the right sinoatrial area and in the uppermost ventricular septum there was a wide myofibrillary injury, similar to contraction band degeneration, typical of hyperacute infarction [25]. Another case of myocardial injury attributable to external cardiac massage in infants has been reported [215].

Compression of the heart between the spine and the sternum exerted during this emergency maneuver causes a direct vertical pressure perpendicular to both the atrial and ventricular septum, which badly stretches the AVN, the bundle of His, and the proximal bundle branches traveling therein [170, 173] (Fig. III.17). The same concept applies to damage to the SAN region, which is located in the vulnerable anatomic junction between the superior vena cava and the thin right atrial wall, and which is associated with the risk of subsequent pacemaker impairment [235]. Such damage could be due to instant cardiac stretching, as well as to prolonged compressive resuscitative maneuvers. Thus, maneuvers involving external cardiac massage, if they are protracted beyond the time limits suggested by recent authoritative criteria [51], may be responsible for the findings of wide myofibrillary injury in the right sinoatrial area and in the uppermost ventricular septum. Such a lesion represents infarct-like damage, as in the patient described above and in many examples of myocardial biopsy [173], following passive instrumental compression and overstretching of the cardiac muscle, that could interfere with the regional contractile activity (Fig. III.18). While stressing that such a maneuver must obviously

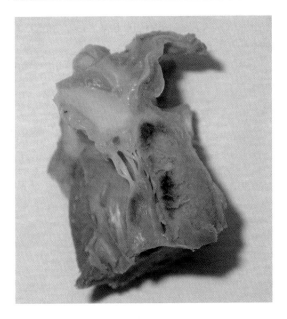

Fig. III.17 During cardiac massage squeezing the heart between the spine and the sternum exerts a direct vertical pressure perpendicular to both the atrial and the ventricular septum. The interventricular septum (block 2 in the study of the cardiac conduction system) has brownish areas attributable to excessive cardiac massage

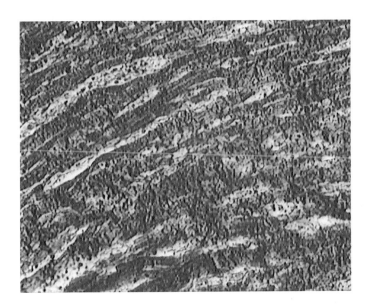

Fig. III.18 Areas of contraction band necrosis in the ventricular septum indicating infarct-like damage (Azan, ×100)

be carried out, we suggest that this should never be prolonged beyond a reasonable time according to the criteria suggested by Eisenberg and Mengert [51].

III.2.18 Coronary Artery Findings

III.2.18.1 Infants

Histological study of the coronary arteries of the 36 SIDS victims examined showed a normal structure in 14. In 22 infants (61%) there was thickening of varying severity in the artery walls. In 11 infants the lesions were initial preatherosclerotic lesions, mostly located in the anterior descending branch of the left coronary artery, while in 11 infants juvenile soft atherosclerotic plaques were observed in all the coronary branches, with narrowing of the lumen (Fig. III.19).

A significant correlation was evident between preatherosclerotic lesions and both formula feeding and parental cigarette smoking (p<0.05). In infants in whom the atherogenic factor was cigarette smoking, especially if the mother was a smoker, the lesions appeared early and were detectable in the first few months of life.

The histological picture varied according to the atherogenic factor. The preatherosclerotic lesions attributable only to the effects of cigarette smoke, observed in five (62%) of the eight breast-fed infants with at least one smoker parent, show an evident structural alteration of the tunica media, which appeared to be fragmented. Marked cell proliferation was also present. The proliferating cells appeared to be arranged in columns with the axis perpendicular to the tunica itself. These elements appeared to infiltrate the intima together with acid mucopolysaccharide deposits, consisting of type A and C chondroitin sulfates and hyaluronic acid, probably synthesized by the smooth muscle cells (SMC) themselves. Low numbers of monocytes were present; B lymphocytes were generally absent.

It should be pointed out that in three breast-fed infants whose parents were non-smokers, preatherosclerotic lesions were present, but soft plaque was not present. Furthermore, in two infants, despite the presence of both atherogenic factors, a normal coronary wall structure was observed [175].

III.2.18.2 Fetuses

Among the 22 fetuses dying suddenly and unexpectedly, no intimal proliferations were revealed by the histological examination of the coronary walls in 10 (45%), but 12 (55%), all of whom died after 35 weeks of gestation, showed multifocal structural alterations of all the coronary arteries, and these were more severe along the anterior descending branch of the left coronary artery. More specifically, in seven of these fetuses (32%), foci of altered architecture of the media with thinning and fiber fragmentation were observed, even in fields far from the bifurcations. The SMCs showed loss of polarity, forming columns of myocytes located perpendicular to the axis of the media itself and infiltrating the subendothelial connective tissue. In five additional fetuses (23%), besides this intense reaction of the SMCs of the media, increased amounts of mucoid ground substance were observed in the subendothe-

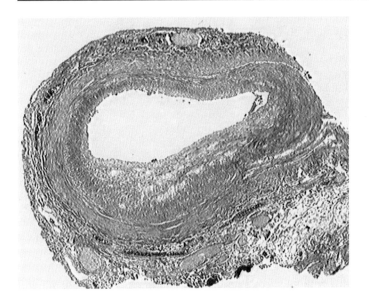

Fig. III.19 Left main coronary artery of a 2-month-old infant dying of SIDS with smoking parents. An early atherosclerotic lesion characterized by soft thickening with numerous foam cells is visible, narrowing the coronary lumen (Azan, ×25)

lial connective tissue, with formation of intimal preatherosclerotic lesions of proliferative aspect (Fig. III.20). Such processes also seem to determine fragmentation and detachment of the internal elastic membrane. Sometimes SMCs appeared in the gaps of this lamina. The clinical data showed that the mothers of 10 of the 12 fetuses with intimal thickenings were smokers before the start of their pregnancy.

In all the lesions, immunohistochemical study of the biological markers showed intense c-fos positivity of the SMCs, while PCNA-positive cells were not detected. The search for chromosome 7 alterations using the FISH technique gave negative results, showing only two normal hybridization spots per nucleus. Frequently, in these cases, apoptotic SMCs were present [139, 179].

A significant correlation ($p<0.05$) was evident between the presence of intimal preatherosclerotic lesions, c-fos gene activation and maternal smoking. Indeed, in 10 of the 12 fetuses of smoker mothers, c-fos-positive preatherosclerotic lesions were present. Only in two fetuses of non-smoking mothers were coronary wall alterations demonstrated [172].

III.2.19 "Gray Zone" or Borderline Cases

III.2.19.1 Cardiac Purkinje Cell Tumor

A 2-month-old female Gypsy infant with no known history of medical problems became unresponsive. The baby was taken to an emergency department where resus-

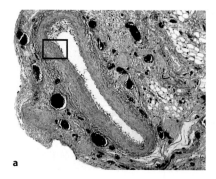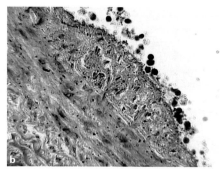

Fig. III.20a,b Left main coronary artery of a fetus of 37 weeks' gestation. The myointimal thickness shows increased amounts of mucoid ground substance in the subendothelial connective tissue (Azan, a ×40, b ×400)

citation was attempted without success until she was pronounced dead 20 minutes after admission. She was born at term, after an uncomplicated pregnancy. No previous ECG recordings were available. Little was known about her family history, since the baby was a Gypsy, and her family moved to another country after her death. Her death remained unexplained after a complete routine autopsy. The case was referred to us at the Institute of Pathology, University of Milan, for more specialized investigations, including study of the cardiac conduction system and brainstem in serial sections.

The heart weighed 46 g, and its dimensions were 4.5×5×3.8 cm in the transverse, longitudinal and anteroposterior directions, respectively. Post-mortem gross cardiac examination revealed cardiomegaly with irregularity of the epicardium (Fig. III.21). On dissection the myocardium was brownish and homogeneous in appearance. The coronary arteries were normally patent [213, 214].

Histological examination of the heart showed nodular aggregates of Purkinje cells throughout the left and right endocardium, the interatrial septum and both the atrial walls. Examination of the conduction system showed the SAN and its adjacent ganglia to be normal. No abnormalities were detected along the internodal pathways. Islands of conduction tissue in the central fibrous body, known as persistent fetal dispersion [205], and areas of resorptive degeneration [88] in the AVN were observed. The complete examination of the cardiac conduction system on serial sections showed the presence of a Purkinje cell tumor near the SAN, and another near the AVN (Fig. III.22). The bundle of His and the bundle branches were unremarkable. The multiple cardiac lesions proved to be small myocardial tumor nodules composed of large cells, characterized by a pale, granular, slightly acidophilic cytoplasm. Cytological atypia was not observed.

The walls of the Purkinje cells varied in thickness and were more dense than those of the normal myocardial cells. In most groups the Purkinje cells were homogeneously distributed, but in some locations they were intermingled with a few other myocardial cells. There was no encasement or capsule about the Purkinje cell

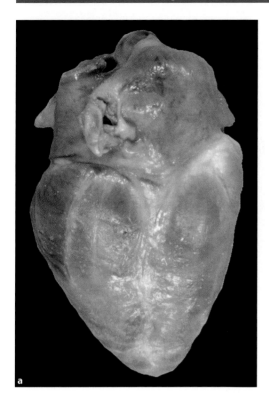
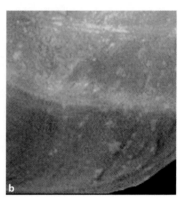

Fig. III.21a,b Cardiac Purkinje cell tumor. **a** Gross cardiac examination reveals generalized cardiac hypertrophy with irregularity of the epicardium. **b** Detail of the epicardium shows the gross aspect of fibrous pericarditis

clusters. The Purkinje cells showed a moderate amount of strongly PAS- and PAS-diastase-positive granular material, typical of glycogen. Only occasional myofibrils were identified within these Purkinje cells. All of the uninvolved myocardial cells were normal in appearance. There was no evidence of myocarditis. The histological examination of the pericardium disclosed a fibrinous pericarditis. The histological examination of the brainstem revealed a mild bilateral hypoplasia of the ARCn. No other significant pathological changes were found.

The Purkinje cell tumors alone may or may not have accounted for the sudden death, but could have played a role in the pathogenesis of the hypoplastic ARCn in this baby [59, 79].

III.2.19.2 Myocardial Infarction and Mahaim Fibers

In a SIDS infant, an accessory Mahaim fiber was associated with acute myocardial infarction. The hypoxia was combined with severe tachycardia (240 beats/minute) due to the accessory Mahaim fiber.

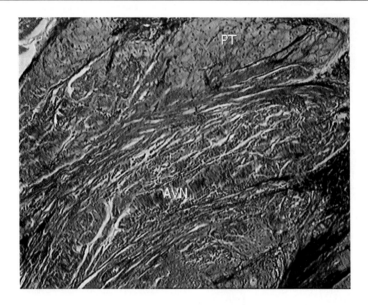

Fig. III.22 Cardiac Purkinje cell tumor. Cluster of Purkinje cells (PT) among normal myocytes, close to the atrioventricular node (AVN) (trichromic Heidenhain, ×100)

III.2.20 Not SIDS/Sudden Explained Death

III.2.20.1 Cardiac Fibroma

A 6-month-old white female with no known history of medical problems, died suddenly and unexpectedly. At autopsy there were no marks of violence. The lungs were congested and slightly edematous. The heart weighed 85 g (expected 31 g), and its dimensions were 6.5 × 7 × 4 cm in the transverse, longitudinal and anteroposterior directions, respectively. Post-mortem gross cardiac examination revealed cardiomegaly with a localized bulge on the anterior left ventricular wall (Fig. III.23a, b). Dissection of the heart showed a mass 4.5 × 4 × 3.5 cm in diameter which completely replaced the ventricular septum and encroached upon the left ventricular chamber, extending from the apex to the base of the heart. The left ventricular cavity, displaced posteriorly, was slit-like. The bulging interventricular septum compressed the infundibulum of the right ventricle. The mass encroached upon and distorted the mitral valve and the aortic outflow. The mass appeared as a single, circumscribed but nonencapsulated lesion; its cut surface was grayish-white, firm and solid and looked trabeculated (Fig. III.23c).

Histological examination of the cardiac tumor showed a nonencapsulated proliferation of fibroblasts with regular nuclei and an abundant network of collagen and elastic fibers that dissociated and entrapped the myocytes. Van Gieson's stain confirmed the presence of collagen fibers which appeared red. These morphological features led to the diagnosis of primary cardiac fibroma [204]. Mitotic figures and

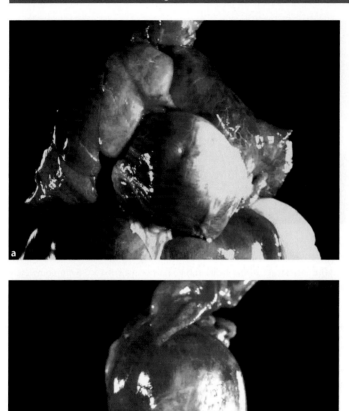

Fig. III.23a–c Explained sudden death caused by cardiac fibroma in a 6-month-old female baby.
a, b Gross cardiac examination revealed cardiomegaly. **c** *see next page*

cytological atypia were not observed. No foci of dystrophic calcification were present. The periphery of the tumor was more cellular and vascular, showing a sparse chronic inflammation basically comprising monocytes. The SAN, adjacent nerve plexuses and the internodal right atrial myocardium were free of alterations. Due to the gross thickening of the interventricular septum due to the tumor, the AVN and its atrial approaches were overstretched horizontally, as well as the bundle of His which was localized on the right side of the pars membranacea septi. The bifurcation of the bundle of His was divaricated and located on the left side of the

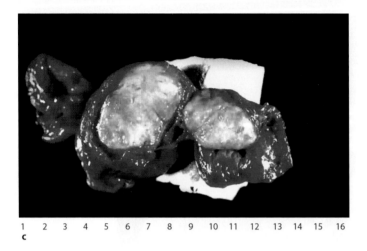

1   2   3   4   5   6   7   8   9   10 11 12 13 14 15 16
c

Fig. III.23a–c *(continued)* **c** Dissection of the heart showed a mass 4.5 × 4 × 3.5 cm completely replacing the ventricular septum, extending from the apex to the base

septal crest. Both bundle branches were found to be compressed. The tumor did not infiltrate the conduction system, which was severely crushed together at the tumor periphery. Sparse chronic inflammation was present at the junction of the tumor and in the common uninvolved myocardium.

III.2.20.2 Hypertrophic Cardiomyopathy

In some cases submitted to our institute with the clinical suspicion of SIDS, a hypertrophic cardiomyopathy, complicated by ischemia or myocardial infarction, has been detected (Fig. III.24).

III.3 Central and Autonomic Nervous System Findings

In SIDS victims, while the gross examination of the brain may not show any alterations, the histopathological study of the autonomic nervous system may show the following frequent congenital anomalies: hypertrophic dendritic spines, hypoplasia/aplasia of the ARCn, and hypoplasia of the reticular formation [181, 190]. The developmental abnormalities associated with SIDS include long dendritic spines, a marker of neuronal immaturity, hypoplasia and agenesis of the brainstem nuclei [178, 181] (Figs. III.25 and III.26).

III.3.1 Hypoplasia and Agenesis of the Arcuate Nucleus

In SIDS, mono- or bilateral hypoplasia, or even agenesis, of the ARCn is particularly frequent. It was observed and studied morphometrically in 56.06% of our cases,

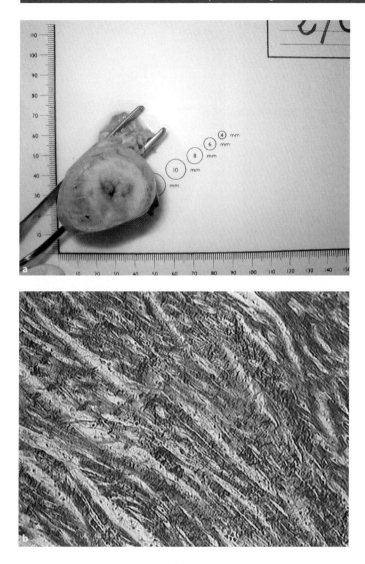

Fig. III.24a,b Explained sudden death in a 3-month-old boy. Massive left ventricular hypertrophy and dyschromic areas (**a**) in the ventricles and septum which was found (**b**) to be areas of contraction band degeneration (Azan, ×100)

and was found to be bilateral diffuse in 26%, bilateral partial (two-thirds caudal) in 17.9%, and monolateral (right) in 12.16% [133, 163, 238].

ARCn hypoplasia has also been detected in 43.3% of stillborns [167, 171, 174, 190, 248]. Morphometric reconstruction allows the volume reduction and the neuronal depletion resulting from this abnormality to be quantified [133, 163]. In every brainstem analyzed, the cytoarchitectural and dimensional parameters of the ARCn

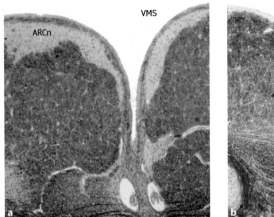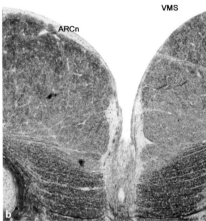

Fig. III.25a,b Sections of the brainstem showing the arcuate nucleus (ARCn) (a) in a 5-month-old infant as control and (b) in a 5-month-old SIDS victim with hypoplasia (VMS ventral medullary surface; Klüver-Barrera, ×25)

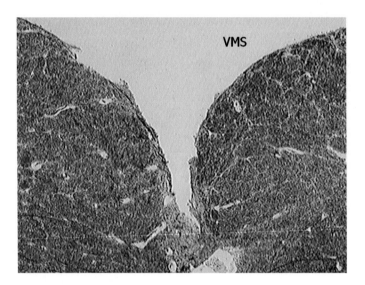

Fig. III.26 Section of the brainstem showing agenesis of the arcuate nucleus in a SIDS victim, an infrequent finding (VMS ventral medullary surface; Klüver-Barrera, ×25)

were compared with those of the nearby olivary nucleus, since both these nuclei have the same embryological origin, arising from the basal lamina of the neuronal tube. The morphometric analysis was performed on serial sections with an image analyzer (Media Cybernetics, Silver Spring, MD, USA) evaluating the mean neuronal density (number of neurons per unit area, expressed as means±SEM millimeters squared) and the mean section area of the neuronal cell bodies (expressed as means±SEM microns squared). We further considered the shape of the cell body, nucleus and nucleolus [212].

In control fetuses under the 25th week of gestation, the ARCn showed a high density of small undifferentiated neuroblasts, which were roundish and apolar with compact chromatin, a nucleolus not clearly identifiable, and scarce cytoplasm (mean cell density 246±14/mm^2, mean cell body area 18±26 μm^2). From the 28th to the 36th week of gestation, the neurons in the ARCn showed a polygonal aspect, and were bipolar with a big vesicular nucleus with loose chromatin (mean density 195±22/mm^2, mean cell area 42±18 μm^2). After birth, the neurons, often multipolar, were decreased in number (mean cell density 140±30/mm^2). The nuclei were enriched with finely scattered chromatin and an evident nucleolus (mean cell body area 81±8 μm^2). The same neuronal model of differentiation was found in the brainstem of SIDS victims with or without ARCn hypoplasia. In the 20% of SIDS victims with normal ARCn architecture an increase in neuronal density was observed (mean value 188±21/mm^2), with smaller neurons (mean neuronal body area 28±20 μm^2). Many of these were lengthened, with a flattened nucleus, compact chromatin, and a poorly evident nucleolus [168].

III.3.2 Combined Pulmonary and Arcuate Nucleus Hypoplasia

In 65% of stillbirths a bilateral pulmonary hypoplasia was observed, characterized by a decrease in volume and/or weight of the lungs, without lobulation anomalies, alteration of the indices of pulmonary development, with a LW/BW ratio below 0.022, a RAC index below 2.2 (Fig. III.27) and the presence of cartilaginous bronchi up to the distal peripheral level. In 31% of cases, a microscopic examination of serial sections of the brainstem showed varying degrees of hypoplasia of the ARCn associated with the simultaneous presence of pulmonary hypoplasia. A significant correlation (p<0.05) between pulmonary hypoplasia and ARCn agenesis/hypoplasia was found [171].

III.3.3 Parabrachial/Kölliker-Fuse Complex Findings

We observed that the morphology of the parabrachial/Kölliker-Fuse (PB/KF) was homogeneous in all cases; therefore we defined the precise structure of the three nuclei [129]. The nucleus of the Kölliker-Fuse is made up of an area of clustered neurons (subnucleus compactus) and an adjacent area with dispersed neurons (subnucleus dissipatus) [190].

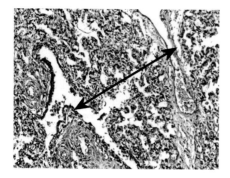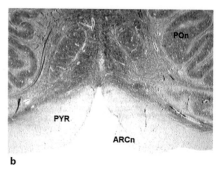

Fig. III.27a,b Combined pulmonary and arcuate nucleus hypoplasia in a SIUD fetus at 39 weeks of gestation. **a** Hypoplastic lung. The black line illustrates the method for determining the radial alveolar count (RAC) (H&E, ×100). **b** Medulla oblongata with severe hypoplasia of the arcuate nucleus (ARCn) (PYR pyramid, POn principal inferior olivary nucleus; Klüver-Barrera, ×25)

III.3.3.1 Morphological Analysis of the Parabrachial/Kölliker-Fuse Complex

Comparative analysis of the serial histological sections obtained from the pons and mesencephalon of the SIUD and SIDS victims with those of the two control groups, made it possible to define the morphological features of the three principal nuclei of the human PB/KF complex: the lateral parabrachial nucleus (lPB), the medial parabrachial nucleus (mPB) and the Kölliker-Fuse nucleus (KF). The PB/KF complex is located in the dorsolateral region of the rostral pons. Only the KF continues along the upper side in the caudal portion of the mesencephalon [132, 136].

III.3.3.2 Lateral Parabrachial Nucleus

In transverse sections this nucleus is located between the lateral surface of the superior cerebellar peduncles (SCP) and the lateral lemniscus. It extends rostrocaudally from the level of the pons–mesencephalon junction (cranial pole) to the level where the lateral nucleus lemniscus is clearly visible (caudal pole). The section marking the passage from the pons to the mesencephalon is recognizable because the SCP forms a continuous line with their decussation. In the more caudal sections, the lPB is reduced because the distance between the lateral lemniscus and the SCP is very short. The neurons are round or tapering, with a light, often central nucleus, a prominent nucleolus, and scarce cytoplasm. Many neurons are dorsoventrally oriented, parallel to the axis of the SCP.

III.3.3.3 Medial Parabrachial Nucleus

This nucleus lies medial to the SCP in transverse sections, running between the motor nucleus of the trigeminal nerves and the locus coeruleus up to the ventral termination of the SCP. Longitudinally, its size does not change from the rostral pole (pons–mesencephalon junction) to the caudal pole (where the lateral nucleus lemniscus is clearly visible). It contains numerous oval and polygonal neurons, which are usually larger than the lPB neurons and have a darker and more evident cytoplasm.

III.3.3.4 Kölliker-Fuse Nucleus

This extends from the caudal pole of the parabrachial nuclei in the rostral pons along the whole of the lower portion of the mesencephalon, up to the level where the caudal pole of the red nucleus is visible.

In transverse pontine sections, it appears as a group of large neurons, located ventral to the lPB, between the medial limit of the SCP and the medial lemniscus. The neurons, which are noticeably larger than those of the PB nuclei, have a large, distinct, eccentric nucleus with a very evident nucleolus, abundant cytoplasm with Nissl substance located at the cell periphery.

On the basis of the neuronal disposition, it is possible at all levels to define two KF subnuclei: the subnucleus compactus, made up of a cluster of a few neurons, whose outline is sometimes indistinct, and the subnucleus dissipatus, adjacent to the compactus. In more rostral sections, in the caudal mesencephalon, the KF, located between the lateral limit of the SCP decussation and the medial lemniscus, shows similar cytological features and neuronal distribution.

III.3.3.5 Morphometric Analysis of the Parabrachial/Kölliker-Fuse Complex

All the morphometric parameters were very similar in SIUD and SIDS victims to those in the respective control groups, as shown by the absence of statistically significant differences between the fetus and infant groups.

The transverse areas and volumes of the PB and KF nuclei in the stillbirth groups (SIUD and stillborn controls) were very frequently lower than those of the infants (SIDS and infant controls); instead, the number of neuronal cells and the cell body areas in fetuses were on the whole larger than in infants, but the differences were not significant.

The coronal size of the lPB decreased from the cranial (total mean area in the four groups 11.29 ± 0.20 mm^2) to the caudal pole (total mean area 2.15 ± 0.28 mm^2). In contrast, the transverse sectional areas of both mPB and KF were similar at the lower and upper extremities (mPB, total mean rostral area 9.28 ± 0.26 mm^2, total mean caudal area 8.55 ± 0.35 mm^2; KF, total mean rostral area 1.75 ± 0.47 mm^2, total mean caudal area 1.88 ± 0.25 mm^2).

Comparing the sectional areas of the body of the three PB/KF nuclei, it was evident that the mPB neurons were larger than the lPB neurons (total mean areas 310.58 ± 0.28 and 268.70 ± 0.36 μm^2, respectively) and that the neuronal areas of the KF were significantly larger, being more than twice those of the PB neurons (mean 878 ± 0.40 μm^2) [132].

In an infant born by cesarian section at 41 weeks of gestation with severe signs of asphyxia and dead 20 hours after delivery, rare and immature neurons were observed in the brainstem areas of both lateral and medial PB nuclei together with a total absence of the characteristic neurons of the KF nucleus.

III.3.4 Brainstem Neurons Responding to Hypoxia (c-fos-Positive)

The immunohistochemical labeling of the c-fos protein in the control group was basically negative or very low. In the medulla oblongata of SIDS victims there was a substantial and significant increase in c-fos expression, limited to the dorsal motor vagal nucleus. Indeed, in 60% of SIDS infants we observed positive neurons with strong cytoplasmic staining distributed in the dorsal motor nucleus of the vagal nerve bilaterally (score from ++ to +++). The c-fos-positive cells were consistently found throughout the rostral-intermediate extent of this nucleus. In contrast, in the caudal sections of the dorsal vagal motor nucleus the immunohistochemical staining was negative or limited [131].

A non-significant scattered distribution of a few c-fos-stained neurons was also present in some cases, irrespective of the positivity of the dorsal vagal motor nucleus, in the inferior olive. Other nuclei of the medulla oblongata examined for c-fos immunoreactivity were negative [131].

III.3.5 Combined Cardiac Conduction and Brainstem Study

A combined morphological post-mortem study of the cardiac conduction system and brainstem was performed in 42 SIDS infants and in 12 controls. Mahaim fibers were observed in 16% of the controls and in 17% of the SIDS infants with the ARCn histologically well developed. In contrast, in SIDS infants with ARCn hypoplasia, Mahaim fibers were observed in 50% of those with severe bilateral hypoplasia (Fig. III.28) and in 71% of those with monolateral hypoplasia. Thus, Mahaim fibers were significantly more frequent in SIDS infants with ARCn hypoplasia than in those with a well-developed ARCn (control and other SIDS infants; p<0.005). The resorptive degeneration, cartilaginous metahyperplasia, and dispersion of the bundle of His bundle were statistically unrelated to the presence of ARCn hypoplasia [169].

III.3.6 Gray-Zone/Borderline SIDS

On the basis of the brainstem findings, a few of our SIDS infants were classified as gray-zone SIDS [214, 273]:

- Case 1: On serial sections the brainstem showed a discrete T-lymphocytic leptomeningitis of the ventral medullary surface, with involvement of the ARCn [159].
- Case 2: On serial sections the brainstem showed toxoplasma encephalitis involving the ambiguous nucleus.
- Case 3: On serial sections the brainstem showed degeneration (of unknown cause, perhaps viral) with a necrotic focus with breaking of nerve fibers into the nucleus of the solitary tract.

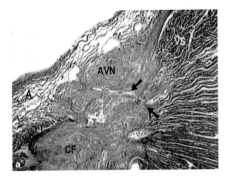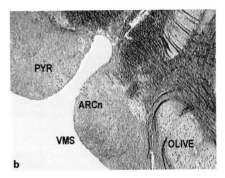

Fig. III.28a,b Simultaneous presence of Mahaim fiber and arcuate nucleus hypoplasia in a SIDS infant. **a** Accessory Mahaim fiber (arrows) bridge the atrioventricular node (AVN) and the ventricular septum (VS) (A right atrium, CF central fibrous body; trichromic Heidenhain, ×25). **b** Severe hypoplasia of the arcuate nucleus (ARCn) (VMS ventral medullary surface, PYR pyramid; Klüver-Barrera, ×25)

- Case 4: On serial sections the brainstem showed a benign hemangioendothelioma arising bilaterally from the area postrema invading the medulla oblongata [160].

III.4 Peripheral Autonomic Nervous System Findings

Regarding abnormalities of the peripheral autonomic nervous system, especially those of the cardiac sympathetic innervations, among 100 SIDS victims, we identified 9 with immature neurons in both the upper cervical ganglia, associated with poorly developed capsular cells and neurons with interneuronal argentaffin elements (small intensely fluorescent, SIF, cells), 25 with hyperplasia of the mediastinal paraganglia, 2 with an intracapsular glomus in the left stellate ganglion, and 5 with inflammatory foci in the right stellate ganglion [181].

III.4.1 Paraganglionic Hyperplasia

Hyperplasia of the aorticopulmonary paraganglia (APP) was detected in 25% of SIDS infants. It was not so marked in intercarotid glomera as in the mediastinal glomera [184, 222]. A few, small, discrete lobules showed great enlargement with irregular and elongated profiles. The enlargement of the APP was due in small part to this increase in size of lobules. The cell clusters and cell diameters were not significantly different from those in age-matched controls. Thus, enlargement of the APP involved an increase in the number rather than size of cells, favoring hyperplasia rather than hypertrophy [222–224]. The prominence of dark cells may be superimposed on the histological features of APP hyperplasia. These were distributed diffusely throughout the glomic tissue, exhibiting a compact basophilic cytoplasm, often in strap-like cytoplasmic extensions with an eccentric hyperchromatic nucleus [224].

The APP of the control group were greater in number and size at birth and decreased dramatically during the first year of life [222].

III.4.2 Stellate Ganglion Alterations

Two SIDS infants showed an intracapsular glomus in the left stellate ganglion and five showed inflammatory foci in the right stellate ganglion.

Alterations in the stellate ganglia may lead to asynchronism of the vagal parasympathetic bradycardic activity with a prevalence of left sympathetic tachycardic activity, and a consequent prolongation of the QT time (long QT syndrome) [240].

Discussion

IV

IV.1 Cardiac Conduction Pathology

The involvement of conducting tissue has been for years a controversial issue in the cardiac pathology of crib death. SIDS infants do not show any abnormality of the ordinary myocardium, while the core of the heart, where cardiac rhythm arises and spreads, represents an insight into the solution to the problem. A pathologist may not consider very small lesions in the general myocardium to have any functional significance and, without experience of looking at the cardiac conduction system, may fail to understand how crucially important a lesion with maximal dimensions of 1 mm could be in the cardiac conduction system [210].

In the 1970s several authors focused the study of crib death on the conducting tissue [7, 55, 56, 87, 89, 144]. The most common finding discussed was the postnatal morphogenesis first defined by James as "resorptive degeneration" [87], consisting of areas of degeneration, cell death mainly by apoptosis [95, 98], and replacement fibrosis, beginning about 1 or 2 weeks after birth [95], and being usually completed in the first year of life [87, 88]. James' concept has been confirmed by Ferris [56], Marino and Kane [150], and Rossi and Matturri [236, 238, 277], but the validity of his findings has been questioned by other investigators [5, 144, 269, 272]. Since this finding was present in both groups, the studies were considered by some authors not conclusive and thus abandoned [208]. Despite the cardiac hypothesis of crib death remaining controversial [4], the concept that crib death may be related to lethal cardiac arrhythmias or heart block due to structural conduction abnormalities now seems to be the focus of renewed interest, as well as the occurrence of infantile junctional tachycardia [72, 161, 198, 199, 201, 208, 210, 254, 263, 284].

The morphological post-mortem study of the conducting tissue in all cases of sudden death in infancy is based on the cardiac concept of crib death, which postulates that it could be due to lethal cardiac electrical instability [4, 210]. This study refers to James' original observations concerning postnatal morphological changes that have been described as present in infants dying in the crib death age range who had no morphological abnormalities [87]. This is what James first referred to as "molding and shaping" of the atrioventricular (AV) node and bundle of His (HB), a process never claimed to be unique to crib death but that, on the contrary, must be considered a normal postnatal morphological change [87, 92, 95, 195]. This postnatal morphogenesis is mediated by apoptotic death of myocytes in both the sinus node and the AV junctional tissue [98, 161]. Since there is no associated inflammation or other indicators of necrosis, some authors have considered such changes as normal or harmless. A misunderstanding of this interpretation has come from two directions: first, those who conclude that a "normal" process could not be seen as pathological; and, second, those who are seeking a single or unique abnormality to blame for crib death. The problem here is that it is not correct to say that because something is normal it is not necessarily dangerous. Since we do not all die during these ubiquitous changes, the changes usually are harmless. This seems to be because no additional other stressful events encountered in a baby's life (such as fever, vomiting or diarrhea and electrolytic imbalance) coincided with the period of postnatal morphogenesis. Thus both cell death and otherwise innocuous events are harmless if they occur alone [144, 210].

IV.1.1 Resorptive Degeneration

During human fetal development, the entire cardiac conduction system is essentially in place and almost completed by the end of the first trimester of gestation. Teleologically, one can reason that this becomes a necessity as a fetus grows and distribution of blood within its body can be facilitated by assisting the circulation provided through the maternal placenta. Once this conduction system has been formed and is in place, there are relatively few morphological changes in it until birth. What happens then is a remarkable transformation and, although the general organization remains, the cytological and histological changes are rather dramatic [88, 101, 102].

The AV node and HB undergo a remarkable postnatal morphogenesis, defined by James [87] in 1968 as "resorptive degeneration", consisting of degeneration, cell death and replacement in an orderly programmed way [87, 89, 92, 95, 198]. This term indicates a tidying-up process in which loose strands of surplus conducting tissue are gradually reabsorbed to change the AV node and HB into their more smooth adult configuration [87, 88, 91, 95]. The areas of resorptive degeneration have been described as clusters of young fibroblasts depositing collagen caught in the central fibrous body, sometimes isolated from the "overdeveloped" specialized structures, sometimes adjacent to them, without association of inflammation or massive necrosis or hemorrhage [87, 238].

We observed areas of resorptive degeneration in 97% of SIDS infants and in 75% of controls (Fig. III.6). Statistical analysis showed a significant difference between the two groups (p<0.05). In these resorptive degeneration areas we observed clusters of young fibroblasts depositing collagen caught in the central fibrous body, sometimes isolated from the overdeveloped specialized structures, sometimes adjacent to them [87, 198]. In these areas there was no associated inflammation nor any massive necrosis or hemorrhage. Macrophages were sometimes present adjacent to the small foci of degeneration, acting eventually as scavenger cells [95, 161, 198] (Figs. III.7 and III.8).

As described by James [87], we also detected resorptive degeneration in both SIDS and control infants, but it was significantly more frequent in the former (p<0.05).

James [92] stated that there is no clear correlation between the extent or presence of degeneration and the age at death. Similarly, we found that the presence of resorptive degeneration was not significantly different among age-related subgroups (p>0.05). James, in his original work [87], emphasized that the process is ubiquitous in the infancy period, being a normal phenomenon rather than a pathological one, but that ubiquity cannot be read as synonymous with safety or stability [95, 103]. In fact, it seems that this normal orderly process, if exaggerated, could provoke blocking disruption of the pathway itself, and if defective could leave in place some accessory communications between the AV pathway and the adjacent ordinary myocardium [72, 161, 198, 200, 237].

The studies of James have been confirmed by some [72, 150, 181, 198–200, 236–238], but have been considered not conclusive by others [4, 5, 7, 269, 272]. Davies et al. [45] pointed out that there is no association between resorptive degeneration and sudden infant death, the process being present equally in SIDS and control infants. Valdés-Dapena et al. [272], Anderson et al. [5] and Lie et al. [144] described fetal dispersion of the AV node without evidence of cell death, phagocytosis or replacement fibrosis. Thiene [267] concluded that the search needs to be continued for a better definition of what is normal and what is abnormal in the conduction system of the infant heart. It has to be underlined that the concept of "resorptive degeneration" remains a contentious issue [4, 210]. In a commentary on one of our previous studies [161], Anderson questioned the definition of "resorptive degeneration" itself [4].

IV.1.2 Atrioventricular Node and Bundle of His Dispersion/Septation

The dispersion or septation of the AV node and/or HB is characterized by fragmentation of the main node/bundle within the central fibrous body [103, 181, 238, 264]. The consequences of this alteration should be intrahissian slowing of the conduction rate producing reentrants, increased automaticity, and paroxysmal block due to fractionation of transmission of the impulse, ventricular arrhythmias and sudden death [101–103, 264].

Dispersion or septation of the HB was observed in 33% of SIDS infants and in 17% of our control infants, without a statistically significant difference (p>0.05) (Fig. III.8). Being present in both groups, therefore, we concur with Suàrez-Mier and Aguilera [263] that HB dispersion cannot be implicated as an unequivocal cause of crib death. Ho and Anderson [83] found HB dispersion and molding in a higher proportion of hearts from controls than from infants dying suddenly and unexpectedly.

In the present study, AVN dispersion/septation [161, 199, 210] was present in 7% of SIDS infants, but was not detected in control infants. As for the septate/dispersed HB, we believe that the consequences of this alteration could be a deceleration of the conduction speed with the phenomenon of reentry, increased automaticity, blocking due to the splitting of the transmission of the impulse, ventricular arrhythmias, and sudden death [19, 264].

IV.1.3 Persistent Fetal Dispersion

The islands of conduction tissue in the central fibrous body, designated as persistent fetal dispersion, have been described as islands of the conduction system separated from the AV node and HB, dispersed in the central fibrous body, resembling the normal fetal pattern [91, 103, 264]. It has been suggested by James [93, 101, 102] that such islands could serve as suitable anatomic substrates for reentrant pathways, dissociation of the conduction impulse and paroxysmal tachycardias. If the dispersed fragments are separated from the AV node or HB but remain attached to the crest of the interventricular septum, their cytological content and anatomic location would favor their function as parasystolic foci with either spontaneous or triggered automatic rhythms, and thus they would serve as abnormal foci of automaticity [91, 93].

Islands of conduction tissue in the fibrous body were found in 25% of our SIDS and in 17% of control infants. In these infants we observed islands of conduction system separated from the AVN and HB, dispersed in the central fibrous body, resembling the normal fetal pattern [91, 103, 210, 264] (Fig. III.8). No statistically significant difference was observed between the SIDS and control groups (p>0.05).

Davies et al. [45] and Suàrez-Mier and Gamallo [264] postulated that fetal dispersion and HB fragmentation may be a normal variation present for many years in life, and must not be considered the anatomic substrate for arrhythmias and sudden death without electrocardiographic abnormalities.

IV.1.4 Accessory Pathways

Frequent alterations in the cardiac conduction system are represented by accessory pathways: Mahaim (Fig. III.9), Kent, and James fibers. These fibers, under particular conditions and under autonomic neural stimulation, may underlie potentially lethal arrhythmias. These arrhythmias are generally junctional reentrant in nature, and are actually the most frequent in the fetus and newborn [88, 161, 181, 238].

The accessory AV pathways can play an important role as the pathogenetic background to a significant number of cardioarrhythmogenic SIDS [195, 210]. The uncommonly numerous group of SIDS infants studied exhibited, as unique histopathological evidence, accessory AV communications, which, however, were "silent" at the clinical level, since they lacked ECG-confirmed tachyarrhythmias [161, 247]. Most of the high-risk tachyarrhythmias in early infancy show the typical ECG of a junctional reentry, together with the inherent implications of a potential or actual degeneration into ventricular fibrillation [247].

IV.1.4.1 Mahaim Fibers

Mahaim fibers are specialized accessory pathways connecting the AV junction and the upper ventricular septum [181, 210, 236, 238]. It seems that whenever the physiological process of resorptive degeneration fails or slows down, some peripheral bundles of the conduction system remain connected to the common myocardial tissue of the ventricular septum, configuring the so-called Mahaim fibers [198, 206, 236, 238]. These fibers, under particular conditions and/or neurovegetative stimuli, may cause potentially malignant junctional arrhythmias [198, 210, 238]. They have been previously described in cases of sudden infant death [28, 37, 236, 238, 263]. Buja et al. [28] reported the case of an infant dying of supraventricular tachycardia; his heart showed a Mahaim fiber in the setting of persistent fetal dispersion consistent with an anatomic substrate for a reentry circuit at the AV junction. Suàrez-Mier and Aguilera [263] found Mahaim fibers in 9 of 55 crib death infants (16.36%) and in none of the control infants, and thus postulated that this type of accessory pathway may be responsible for death in some crib death infants. We detected specialized connections between the AV junction and the upper ventricular septum, named Mahaim fibers [161, 181, 236, 238], in 23% of SIDS and in 8% of control infants. The difference between the two groups was not statistically significant (p>0.05) (Fig. III.9). When there is a working accessory AV connection, the whole AV system or its junctional tract, can become part of a classic circuit of a tachycardic macroloop. The preexcitation depends on the presence of AV accessory pathways where the impulse can diffuse in an antegrade direction [19, 181].

IV.1.4.2 Kent Fibers

A defective resorptive degeneration that may rarely result in an accessory pathway between the atrial and ventricular myocardium [181, 236, 238], the classic Kent bundle responsible for the Wolff-Parkinson-White (WPW) syndrome [282], was detected in two of our SIDS infants (2%), but was not found in any of the control infants. It is an accessory pathway that has an arrhythmogenic action, since it provides direct communication between the atrium and the ventricle, bypassing the classic conduction system pathway. This Kent bundle allows the passage of a faster impulse than that continuing in the normal conduction system pathway, since the deceleration of the AVN has been bypassed. This could result in some serious tachyarrhythmias: a ventricular tachycardic preexcitement and atrial retrograde excitement through the Kent bundle. The presence of this bundle does not mean that it necessarily conducts an impulse bypassing the AVN to prematurely excite the HB, since the AVN and HB can conduct the impulse only in a retrograde and/or intermittent way [242]. Moreover, a more rapid conduction in the bypass would produce excitement in the HB before the impulse could reach the ventricle through the AVN; in such a case, a simultaneous diffusion of the impulse both toward the HB, or toward the AVN, could result in fusion of the ventricular complex (delta wave) [242, 282].

IV.1.4.3 James Fibers

James fibers are defined as atriohissian accessory pathways connecting the right atrium directly to the HB [193], and were observed in two SIDS infants (2%) and in none of the control infants.

IV.1.5 Cartilaginous Metahyperplasia

The fibroblasts of the central fibrous body seem to have a pluripotential nature, although the functional meaning of this is still unknown [91, 161]. In normal circumstances they produce dense collagen, but there are examples of cartilage or sometimes bone present in the central fibrous body [57, 103]. It is reasonable that the fibroblasts of the fibrous body, essential to complete the morphogeny of the adjoining AV node and HB, may sometimes work improperly, becoming both hyperactive and inactive. If they are able to produce media different from collagen, they could also show metaplastic transformation. What could induce such metaplasia is completely unknown, although it could logically be suspected that it is a consequence of physical stress, ischemia or other unknown factors [91, 210]. For example, the synthesis of the DNA of the cartilaginous cells is stimulated by oscillating electric fields [109], and it could be supposed that such an effect exists in the fibrous body or near to it [91]. Cartilaginous metahyperplasia of the central fibrous body has already been described in cases of cardiac sudden death [91, 161, 238].

Since the AV node lies directly upon the central fibrous body and the HB courses through it, they both seem to be in some jeopardy because of their proximity when an alteration of the central fibrous body is present [87, 263]. It seems that a central fibrous body with cartilaginous metahyperplasia could potentially have provoked compression of the HB and the conduction system in many crib death infants [232]. Ferris et al. [56] described two infants dying unexpectedly with the post-mortem findings of nodules of fibrocartilage within the central fibrous body adjacent to the HB and AV node. In the present study, we detected cartilaginous metahyperplasia of the central fibrous body [9, 70] in 6% of SIDS infants and in 4% of control infants, without a statistically significant difference ($p > 0.05$) between the two groups (Fig. III.10). James [93] reported that cartilaginous or bony metaplasia in infants suffering sudden and unexpected death originates from the pluripotential fibroblasts of the fibrous body, but their role in causing the death is not yet entirely understood.

IV.1.6 Hemorrhage of the Cardiac Conduction System

Hemorrhage of the conducting tissue is generally considered present when red blood cells are seen in the intercellular spaces [5]. In the present study, hemorrhage of the AV junction was detected only in SIDS infants (16%). In some SIDS infants the red cells were widely dispersed over an area of specialized myocardium, in others discrete clumps of red cells were present enclosing several working as well as specialized myocardial fibers. Since an emergency resuscitation effort was made in almost all of our crib death infants, including external cardiac massage, Rossi et al. [173] considered that the hemorrhage occurred after death, due to injury caused by the attempted resuscitation effort. As we have previously reported [161], it is difficult to distinguish between junctional hemorrhage occurring during life and that occurring immediately after death. Other investigators [5, 144, 263], with a larger number of controls, found hemorrhagic lesions present in both groups. Jankus [108], in his report of three crib death and three explained death cases, found hemorrhage exclusively in the crib death infants.

IV.1.7 Intramural Right Bundle Branch

An intramural right bundle branch was present, respectively, in 20% and 25% of SIDS and control infants, and the difference was not significant (p>0.05). In SIDS infants dying from 3 to 60 days an intramural right bundle was more frequent than in those dying from 61 to 120 days (p=0.01). This finding is not of particular concern since the intramural right bundle is considered a normal variation in the location of the right bundle branch [93, 161].

IV.1.8 Left-Sided Bundle of His

In the present study, a left-sided HB was present in 20.29% of SIDS infants and in 8.3% of explained death infants, without a statistically significant difference. In one infant the HB was left-sided and intramural (Fig. III.12). Bharati et al. [22] observed a left-sided HB significantly more commonly in crib death infants (53.3%) than in explained death infants (25%), suggesting that this may be a factor promoting crib death. Massing and James [154] found a left-sided HB in 62.5% of normal human hearts of various ages. A left-sided HB has been described in association with sudden death in previously healthy individuals [19, 22] and in asthmatics [20].

IV.1.9 Intramural Left Bundle Branch

An intramural left bundle [229] was observed in 2% of SIDS infants and in none of the control infants (Fig. III.6 and III.12). Rossi [229] reported that an intramural left bundle branch is comparatively more vulnerable to an impaired blood supply through the nutrient arteries.

IV.1.10 Septation of the Bifurcation

Septation of the bifurcation, also known as anomalous bifurcation [161, 238], was detected in 13% of SIDS infants but was not found in infants. Thus, if the results in our series are confirmed in other even larger studies, these changes might be responsible for death in some SIDS infants.

IV.1.11 Hypoplasia of the Cardiac Conduction System

SAN hypoplasia [22, 238] was found in 6% of SIDS infants, but was not found in explained death infants (Fig. III.6). Studies of the cardiac conduction system in crib death are usually directed towards the AV node and HB, but it seems that the sinus node may also be involved. Ho et al. [84] described three perinatal infants with a hypoplastic sinus node and cardiac arrhythmia immediately before death. They considered the hypoplasia of the sinus node as due to an arrest or defect in development rather than due to an active degenerative process. Kozakewich et al. [124], examining the sinus node of 30 crib death and 18 explained death infants, found no difference in size between the two groups, but found intimal lesions of the sinus node intranodal artery in three crib death infants.

Hypoplasia of the HB was detected in 5% of our SIDS infants and in none of the control infants (Fig. III.6).

IV.1.12 Atrioventricular Node/Bundle of His Dualism

The AV node and HB show a "dualism" in which they appear stratified into two portions by interposition of a fibrous diaphragm, so configuring the morphological basis of dual AV pathways [161, 201, 241]. AVN dualism [201, 241] was present in 3% of our SIDS infants (Fig. III.14) who died at between 3 and 120 days of life, and in none of the explained death infants. HB dualism was present in 3% of SIDS infants and in 4% of the control infants. In these infants the AVN and/or the HB appeared stratified into two portions by interposition of a fibrous diaphragm [161, 210] (Fig. III.6). Bharati et al. [21] described a distinct AV node-like structure on the parietal wall of the right atrium in a patient with a history of paroxysmal supraventricular tachycardia.

IV.1.13 Zahn Node

The Zahn node [227, 277, 285] is also known as the coronary sinus node because it is situated near the myocardium of the coronary sinus outlet [227]. Doerr [48] in 1957 presented a large illustration of a Zahn node represented as a Y-shaped bundle of loosely arranged myocardial fibers embracing a neurovegetative ganglion and protruding from an "atrial tail" of the AV node, close to the coronary sinus [227]. Doerr and Schiebler [49] recognized that it is difficult to decide whether a coronary sinus node can be considered as a separate entity of the conducting system or only as the dorsal atrial part of the AV node.

A Zahn node was present in 3% of the SIDS infants but in none of the control infants (Fig. III.6). In these infants, close to the major axis of the AVN, a formation of small myocytes, lengthened or stellate in shape, arranged with a muscular network was observed, morphologically definable as a small AVN. A typical feature of a Zahn node is a posterosuperior prolongation with a pseudohissian fascicle. One these cases was previously reported and discussed as a plausible substrate for reentry tachyarrhythmias [158].

IV.1.14 Fibromuscolar Hyperplasia of the Conduction System Arteries

Histological examination of serially sectioned coronary arteries from our infants who died suddenly and unexpectedly revealed the frequent presence of preatherosclerotic lesions, indicating the atherogenic effect of cigarette smoke (Fig. III.19) [175, 177].

Both intrauterine and postnatal exposure to cigarette smoke appear to increase the risk of sudden death in infancy [191]. Nicotine seems to interact directly with the endogenous nicotinic and muscarinic cholinergic receptors present in the brainstem regions involved in cardiorespiratory activity, jeopardizing their normal function in vulnerable subjects.

The consequences of formula feeding are also significant. The 55th World Health Assembly [283] recently recommended breast feeding for at least the first 6 months of life, to avoid the serious damage caused by formula feeding. Unlike formula milk, maternal milk contains long-chain polyunsaturated fatty acids (LCPUFAS), which are necessary for the normal development of several tissues [128]. The coronary and cardiac conduction system artery lesions were larger and more diffuse in formula-fed infants whose parents both smoked. The combination of both risk factors seems to increase the early atherogenic effect of each noxa.

This study stresses the severe and early atherogenic action of both baby formula and cigarette smoke, demonstrable in the cardiac conduction system arteries as well as in coronary walls of infants. The association of the two atherogenic noxae results in a cumulative effect [177].

Fibromuscular hyperplasia or dysplasia [94] of the sinus node and/or AV node arteries has been described as a cause of death in young people and adults [103, 104]. Anderson and Hill [3], analyzing 40 victims of crib death, found 5 infants (12.5%) with increased thickness of the AV artery and one infant with reduced thickness of the sinus node artery. The authors hypothesized that this thickness may explain ischemia of the conducting tissue with consequent cardiac arrhythmias and/or heart block.

We detected early preatherosclerotic lesions of the SAN and/or AVN arteries in 21% of our infants (Fig. III.15). This percentage is much higher than that found by Suàrez-Mier and Aguilera (1.8%) [263] and more similar to that found by Anderson and Hill (12.5%) [3].

These lesions should be regarded as "initial preatherosclerotic lesions" instead of "fibromuscular hyperplasia" or "dysplasia" of the cardiac conduction system arteries [177].

In the cardiac conduction system arteries early atherosclerotic lesions are detectable in early infancy and might have a significant role in determining sudden infant death. Our results suggest the importance of studying suitable strategies for eliminating the risk factors, i.e. parents smoking and formula feeding, thus preventing the development of atherosclerotic lesions [175, 177].

IV.1.15 Apoptosis Expression in the Conducting Tissue

The programmed cell death called apoptosis is of particular interest [44, 85, 99, 100, 162, 251]. Its unpredictable occurrence could play a role in the pathogenesis of crib death [95, 98, 162, 207, 210].

The apoptotic indices (AI) in the cardiac conduction system of SIDS infants (range 0.80–4.50, mean±SEM 2.45±0.44) and of controls (range 2.79–3.00, mean±SEM 2.89±0.05) were found to show no statistically significant difference (p>0.05, Student's t test), while in the resorptive degeneration areas the AI was higher in the controls than in the SIDS infants (p<0.05, Student's t test). The SAN in both groups showed an AI similar to that of the common myocardium. The AI was higher in the AVN, HB and the initial tract of the bundle branches than in the common myocardium (p<0.05, Student's t test) [162, 207]. In almost all cases, TUNEL labeling was detected in the peripheral region of the AVN, close to the atrial myocardium (Fig. III.16). This is in agreement with the observations of James [90] who reported that the AV node, during postnatal morphogenesis, becomes smaller towards its adult configuration, being reabsorbed mainly at its periphery and almost always along its left margin, and that apoptosis is a major and possibly the main mechanism by which cell death occurs during the postnatal morphogenesis of the cardiac conduction system [95].

The postnatal morphogenesis of the sinus node by apoptosis occurs generally in the same time period (first year of life) as the postnatal morphogenesis of the AV node and HB. This involves multifocal cell death by apoptosis and could serve to distort further the normal rhythm of the baby's heart. While the changes in the AV node and HB are mainly smoothing of the margins of these two structures, eliminating surplus tissue that may be dangerous if not removed, the changes in the sinus node are quite different, amounting more or less to a total restructuring of the interior of the sinus node itself. The fetus and the infant have sinus nodes composed primarily of P cells, whereas the sinus node of the adult human always contains a mixture of slender cells and P cells. The changes occur either by transformation of some of the P cells to slender cells or by the death of P cells to be replaced by slender cells, perhaps migrating in from the margins of the sinus node [95, 98]. Cardiac arrhythmias, such as atrial fibrillation or atrial flutter, as well as distortions in sinus rhythm, including episodes of sinus arrest or tachycardia or ectopic beading, are facilitated by impaired activity of the sinus node during its molding [162, 237].

It has been suggested that apoptosis of the cardiac conduction system could be a process favoring electrical instability in two opposite ways. Defective apoptosis could leave in place some accessory communication between the AV pathway and the adjacent ordinary myocardium, and would leave the sinus node in its fetal configuration, eliminating the beneficial evolution into an appropriate mixture and distribution of P cells among slender cells [18, 95, 198, 210]. Exaggerated apoptosis, could provoke blocking disruption of the pathway itself, and disfigure the sinus node structure or even completely destroy it [95, 106, 107, 238]. Kajstura et al. [114], in their study of programmed cell death during cardiac maturation in rats, found that myocyte death is absent in the fetal heart but affects the myocardium postnatally, particularly the right ventricle.

IV.1.16 PCNA Expression in the Conducting Tissue

Although many experimental cell kinetic studies have demonstrated that the number of proliferating myocytes in the mammalian heart is high during embryogenesis, but gradually decreases becoming similar to a "non-dividing" tissue [15, 151, 249], the findings of several studies [8, 249] and of a study by us [203] show that, in some pathological conditions, myocardial cells are still able to express PCNA and nuclear mitotic division. This prompted us to hypothesize that during postnatal cardiac molding the cell death could be accompanied by cell proliferation. However, in the present study, in both the SIDS and the control groups there were no findings of positive PCNA immunoreactivity either in the conducting system or in the common myocardium. Kajstura et al. [114] found that in rats the DNA synthesis in myocytes decreases postnatally with maturation.

IV.1.17 ECG Findings

One or more electrocardiograms were available in 15% of our SIDS infants, but in our infants a more careful clinicopathological and electrocardiographic correlation still remains to be done. Schwartz et al. [254], in their prospective study, performed follow-up ECG in an unselected population of 33,034 infants. They found that prolongation of the QT interval in the first week of life is strongly associated with SIDS [254]. However, Schwartz et al. did not perform a post-mortem morphological study in the SIDS cases, which is considered of great importance by other authors [21, 96, 105, 240]. In particular, James [96] studied in detail the pathophysiological significance of conduction system morphological abnormalities in long QT (LQT) syndrome.

IV.1.18 Coronary Artery Findings

IV.1.18.1 Infants

Histological examination of serially sectioned coronary arteries from 36 SIDS victims revealed the frequent presence (61% of infants) of initial atherosclerotic lesions, indicating the atherogenic effect of passive cigarette smoke.

The severity of the lesions ranged from initial preatherosclerotic alterations, mainly affecting the anterior descending branch of the left coronary artery, observed in 11 infants, to juvenile soft plaques, which can be so extensive as to reduce the arterial lumen by up to 30–40%. These soft plaques were observed in all the coronary walls in 11 infants.

The morphological appearance of the preatherosclerotic lesions varies in relation to the type of atherogenic noxa. In infants in whom the atherogenic factor is related exclusively to cigarette smoke, particularly if the mother smoked before becoming pregnant, the lesions can usually be detected very early, within the first few months of life.

Another notable feature is the structural disorder of the tunica media, which appears to be fragmented and is also the site of intense proliferation. The myointimal thickening consists predominantly of smooth muscle cell (SMC) infiltrates, rare monocytes and B lymphocytes. The deposits of amorphous material, which contribute to the myointimal thickening, are made up of acid mucopolysaccharides (Fig. III.19).

Both intrauterine and postpregnancy exposure to cigarette smoke appear to increase the risk of SIDS [191]. Nicotine seems to interact directly with the endogenous nicotinic and muscarinic cholinergic receptors present in the brainstem regions involved in cardiorespiratory activity, jeopardizing their normal function in vulnerable subjects [119].

The consequences of formula feeding may also be significant. The 55th World Health Assembly [283] recently recommended breast feeding for at least the first 6 months of life, to avoid the serious damage caused by formula feeding. Unlike formula milk, maternal milk contains LCPUFAS, which are necessary for the normal development of many tissues [128]. The positive effects of breast feeding have also been demonstrated with regard to SIDS, whose incidence is lower in breastfed infants [68].

The coronary lesions were larger and more diffuse in formula-fed infants whose parents both smoked. The combination of both risk factors seems to increase the atherogenic effect of each noxa. The association of the two atherogenic noxae appears to have a cumulative effect and leads to the early development of typical atherosclerotic plaques [175].

IV.1.18.2 Fetuses

We have analyzed the morphological pattern of preatherosclerotic coronary artery lesions in human fetuses and the possible atherogenic role of maternal cigarette smoking before and during pregnancy [172].

In the literature, the few studies carried out on fetal coronary arteries have predominantly been performed in experimental animals. Bolande et al. [24] observed that proliferative modifications of the coronary arteries are present in 100% of piglet fetuses and regress after birth, and they conclude that such lesions represent a physiological developmental process and therefore cannot be related to coronary atherogenesis in the adult.

The rare studies of the coronary arteries of human fetuses in the literature yield controversial findings and date back over 30 years. In a study in 1957 [189], Moon did not observe any pathological process, while a few years later, Robertson [226] reported an altered architecture of the coronary walls only in fetuses at term.

The results of our histopathological study performed on the major epicardial coronary arteries, serially sectioned, from 22 late stillborns, have enabled us to demonstrate the incidence and characteristics of intimal preatherosclerotic lesions of proliferative appearance and the possible role of maternal cigarette smoking. In particular, our findings show that at first the intima appears to be infiltrated by SMCs which, due to loss of polarity, seem to be arranged in a column perpendicular to the main axis of the media. The longitudinally oriented SMCs probably originate from the media but they are intimal structures. Only later does the intimal thickening contain acid mucopolysaccharide deposits, probably synthesized by SMCs, that give an edematous appearance to the subendothelial connective tissue. Few monocytes are present (Fig. III.20). These intimal preatherosclerotic lesions of proliferative appearance were observed in 12 stillborns, 10 of whose mothers were smokers.

Molecular biology analyses in our study have made it possible to clarify the biological nature of the observed coronary wall alterations observed. These studies revealed intense activation of the protooncogene c-fos, while proliferative PCNA expression and trisomy of chromosome 7 were not observed. Frequently, in these cases, apoptotic SMCs were present [11, 139].

The c-fos gene belongs to the family of immediate early genes, so defined for their ability to be rapidly activated in many tissues in response to various injuries, because they do not require protein synthesis. Therefore, c-fos positivity in fetal coronary lesions represents the first biological reaction in response to the gaseous products of nicotine combustion. By crossing the cellular membrane, particularly of the SMCs, the nicotine products can directly modify the expression of the c-fos gene, interacting with nuclear receptors [139].

We have demonstrated that very early preatherosclerotic alterations of the coronary arteries are already detectable in the prenatal period and are significantly associated with maternal cigarette smoking even before the beginning of pregnancy [172].

IV.1.19 "Gray Zone" or Borderline Cases

Of particular interest are borderline SIDS infants whose microscopic examination showed specific lesions interacting with the conduction system. In particular, a multifocal Purkinje tumor near the AV node [213, 214]. What makes this case unique and a "borderline case" is the combination of a multifocal nodular Purkinje tumor of the heart associated with a bilateral hypoplasia of the arcuate nucleus (ARCn). The Purkinje cell tumor alone may have or may not have accounted for the sudden death, but could have played a triggering role in this baby suffering from a hypoplastic ARCn. This case seems in part consistent with the triple-risk model of crib death, a hypothesis that invokes underlying biological vulnerability to exogenous stressors or triggering factors in a critical developmental period [59, 179]. Further studies on triggering factors and related mechanisms will lead to a better understanding of the complex interactions involved in the pathophysiology of crib death [213, 214].

Accessory fibers, under particular conditions and under autonomic neural stimulation, may underlie potentially lethal arrhythmias. These arrhythmias are generally junctional reentrant in nature, being actually the most frequent in the fetus and newborn [284]. Severe oxygen-consuming tachycardias can underlie, in hypoxic infants, the risk of myocardial infarction.

IV.1.20 Other Cardiac Findings

In some cases submitted to our institute with the clinical suspicion of SIDS, an explained cardiac cause of death was identified, i.e. a cardiac fibroma, and several cases of hypertrophic cardiomyopathy, complicated with ischemia or myocardial infarction (Figs. III.23 and III.24).

Recently, Valdés-Dapena and Gilbert-Barness [270] have pointed out that cardiac causes for sudden infant death include viral myocarditis, congenital heart disease particularly congenital aortic stenosis, endocardial fibroelastosis, and anomalous origin of the left coronary artery from the pulmonary artery. Other cardiac conditions that may result in sudden death include rhabdomyomas of the heart in tuberous sclerosis and conduction system disorders. Frequent conduction system disorders resulting in sudden death include histiocytoid cardiomyopathy, congenital heart block that may be associated with maternal lupus erythematosus, arrhythmogenic right ventricular dysplasia, and LQT syndromes [270].

IV.2 Neuropathology

Among the most important pathogenetic theories of SIDS (respiratory, cardiac, and visceral dyskinetic) the congenital and acquired abnormalities of the central nervous system, particularly of the brainstem (Figs. III.23 and III.24), are attracting the greatest interest [132].

IV.2.1 Hypoplasia and Agenesis of the Arcuate Nucleus

In SIDS mono- or bilateral hypoplasia or even agenesis of the ARCn was found to be particularly frequent, as it occurred in over 50% of our SIDS infants (Figs. III.23 and III.24).

The ARCn is a bulbar chemosensitive nucleus which takes part in the regulation of cardiorespiratory activity [58, 118, 133, 163, 167, 238]. This anatomic site, relevant to the central cardiopulmonary hypothesis in SIDS and SIUD, is located near the surface of the ventrolateral, ventral, and ventromedial medulla oblongata [174]. This region is an integrative site for autonomic function, ventilation, and chemosensitivity. It contains sympathetic premotor pressor and depressor zones which regulate blood pressure, cardiac rate and rhythm, and hemodynamic aspects of temperature regulation, as well as neurons which integrate "defense" responses [58].

A high frequency of hypoplasia of the ARCn occurs in fetuses who died "sine causa" (SIUD) in a similar manner to that observed in SIDS, as well as in newborns who died suddenly and unexpectedly [135, 140, 167, 171, 174, 190, 248].

Our study of ARCn cellular maturation suggests that in some SIDS infants even an architecturally well-developed ARCn could have a pattern of anomalous neuronal differentiation. Such a maturation defect may be related to developmental disorders of the ARCn chemoreceptor function and consequently to respiratory regulation impairment [212].

Cigarette smoking was significantly associated with structural alterations of the ARCn (bilateral hypoplasia, monolateral hypoplasia, partial hypoplasia, delayed neuronal maturation, decreased neuronal density) [133].

IV.2.2 Combined Pulmonary and Arcuate Nucleus Hypoplasia

Using specific macro- and microscopic criteria, we have also demonstrated the presence of pulmonary hypoplasia in a high percentage of stillbirths (65%). In 31% of fetuses the lung hypoplasia was associated with hypoplasia of the medullary ARCn (Fig. III.27) [171]. This suggests that in these cases hypoplasia of the ARCn exerts a negative effect on respiratory movements in utero and therefore on lung development. In fetuses in which pulmonary hypoplasia is not accompanied by hypodevelopment of this nucleus the explanation could be a wrong physiological mechanism, more precisely a failure to block the inhibitory action on the Kölliker-Fuse nucleus exerted by the gigantocellular nucleus.

Fetal respiration appears to be a feature of mammalian development, even though it has been studied in detail only in sheep. In their original study, Dawes et al. [46] describe in the fetal lamb rapid and irregular breathing movements alternating with apneic pauses of varying duration, very long in the early stages of gestation and reducing gradually thereafter in relation to pulmonary development, irrespective of the gas profile of the blood.

Experimental physiological studies have shown that the predominant absence of ventilation in utero is determined by the inhibitory effect exerted mainly by the Kölliker-Fuse nucleus. In the fetus there is periodic disinhibition of the Kölliker-Fuse nucleus to allow breathing movements which favor pulmonary development. This interruption of inhibitory activity seems to be determined by a nucleus located in the caudal portion of the pons, the gigantocellular nucleus, which after birth has the task of intervening rhythmically to interrupt the inhibitory effect on inspiration normally exerted by the Kölliker-Fuse nucleus, and enabling expiration to start [171].

Developments in magnetic resonance imaging have recently led to the possibility of analyzing the development of specific fetal structures in utero and therefore to the ability to diagnose both ARCn and lung hypoplasia prenatally [171]. This has provided a number of potentially clinically useful applications, and allows prenatal counseling and therapeutic planning.

IV.2.3 Parabrachial/Kölliker-Fuse Complex Findings

The parabrachial/ Kölliker-Fuse (PB/KF) complex has been defined in different animal species as lying in the dorsolateral part of the pontine tegmentum and is subdivided into three well-defined regions: the medial parabrachial (mPB) nucleus, the lateral parabrachial (lPB) nucleus, and the Kölliker-Fuse (KF) nucleus. Experimental studies have demonstrated that the PB/KF complex is involved in a variety of functional activities and plays an important role in respiratory activity. In humans, the impossibility of using experimental approaches makes it difficult to characterize the cytoarchitecture and the physiology of these structures. Only a few studies have provided morphological data regarding the human PB complex, but these data are imprecise and conflicting [36, 82, 132, 136].

Our brainstem findings confirm the hypothesis that functional or structural alterations of components of the vegetative nervous system which modulate fetal breathing may lead to disturbances in the development of the respiratory apparatus, in particular to pulmonary hypoplasia in stillbirth [165, 171]. Although irrelevant to fetal life, the chemoreceptors become of vital importance in the intrapartum and postpartum periods; therefore, when they are impaired in development, they may underlie cardioventilatory abnormalities critical to SIDS [79, 134, 137, 165].

A relevant question concerns how this congenital anomaly may cause respiratory disturbances immediately after birth, as suggested by the examination of a well-documented intrapartum case in our series. In this infant, an anomalous position of the umbilical cord could have enhanced a chemoreceptor dysfunction and this may have been an important predisposing or contributing lethal factor. Respiratory insufficiency was seen immediately, a fact that seems to indicate that the pathogenetic mechanism of respiratory death involves two factors: (1) vulnerability due to hypoplasia of the ARCn, and (2) an exogenous stress represented by the trauma of birth.

Chemoreceptors are normally well developed in late pregnancy, but not yet functioning do not interfere with the intrauterine survival of the fetus itself. These same central and peripheral receptors will, however, be ready for their correct chemoreflexogenic function upon delivery as soon as the blood circulation shifts from the maternal–fetal oxygenation to the newborn's respiratory breathing, which is sharply divergent from the former. Moreover, this novel chemoreceptor-dependent breathing contrasting with the fetal oxygen supply, may make a developmental chemoreceptor functional impairment manifest itself only during the intrapartum or postpartum periods, with obvious, yet unpredicted, ominous sequelae. This ill-understood reflex-blocking center, exerting in the fetus the life-preserving disfacilitation of the inhibitory action upon chemoreflexes, has been broadly localized in animal experiments to the lateral cranial pons near the branching of the upper cerebellar pedunculi, so deserving the toponym "parabrachial" Kölliker-Fuse complex. This nuclear area, in the near-term fetus accounts for the strong inhibitory action of chemoreflexogenesis that prevents potentially lethal active respiratory motions in the fetus. During a still-indefinite phase of partum, the Kölliker-Fuse nucleus quickly reverses to an active respiration-facilitating function, and it is then actually regrouped among the respiratory centers in postnatal physiology. A new possibility, as yet poorly investigated, suggests that not only abnormalities of the respiratory chemoreceptors may underlie SIDS by defective regulation, but also anomalous persistence of post-partum blockade or disfacilitation of respiratory fetal chemoreflexes may play a part in the respiratory, life-threatening mechanisms of SIDS itself [79, 165].

IV.2.4 Brainstem Neurons Responding to Hypoxia (c-Fos-Positive)

Immunohistochemistry of c-fos applied to the medulla oblongata of SIDS victims has shown that in 60% of SIDS infants there is a high density of labeled neurons in the dorsal motor vagal nucleus [131]. The cellular changes induced by increased Fos protein in the dorsal motor vagal nucleus neurons are still unclear. In many proliferative processes, particularly during embryonic development and in some types of tumors [50], the rapid activation of the c-fos gene in the presence of different noxae causes activation of other genes related to DNA synthesis. This mitogenic effect does not occur in the nerve cells. The increased Fos expression in the dorsal motor vagal nucleus neurons observed in this study could enhance the production of catecholamines, indispensable for the breathing stimuli [131]. Although the functioning of the c-fos gene remains poorly understood, the increase in fos immunoreactivity observed in our SIDS infants suggests that the neurons of the dorsal motor nucleus of the vagal nerve involved in breathing regulation may yield an intense, immediate ventilatory response to hypoxia [131].

IV.2.5 Gray Zone/Borderline SIDS

Inflammatory brainstem lesions, sometimes of suspected viral origin, are significant. Particularly interesting is our observation of a 4-month-old infant with dysfunction in autonomic cardiorespiratory regulation. The infant had a T-lymphocytic leptomeningitis affecting the ventral medullary surface, with involvement of the outer layer of a hypoplastic ARCn. This case illustrates the etiopathogenetic importance of a combined lesion of the central chemosensitive field [225]. Focal degeneration and necrosis of the solitary nucleus was observed in another case. Such a clinically ignored infection might have simultaneously compromised respiratory and cardiac activity, together with the kinesis of the tongue, glottis, esophagus and/or stomach. In particular, a lingual/glottic kinetic problem might have compromised the tone of the tongue, with the risk of high respiratory obstruction in the supine position, besides provoking glottic spasm and/or inspiration of gastroesophageal reflux [79].

Recent studies on the pathophysiology of SIDS have focused on the cardiorespiratory brainstem of infants, with important results pointing to a reflexogenic lethal mechanism [58, 118]. We examined the case of a 4-month-old male, who suffered from deglutition and respiratory disorders. On post-mortem investigation a hemangioendothelioma was identified in the area postrema, which widely infiltrated the posterior–middle brainstem bilaterally, sparing only the dorsal vagal nucleus, while diffusely compromising, even cancelling, the neuronal circuitries of the hypoglossus, solitary tract, ambiguous nucleus, and the reticular formation [160]. It was evident that the baby survived 4 months because of preservation of the chemosensitive respiratory ventral medullary surface areas together with the ARCn, and the dorsal visceromotor nucleus. All our observations confirm the pathological evidence and the inherent clinical implications, focused upon the brainstem cardiovascular and respiratory centers, whose derangement can trigger SIDS [79].

The inflammatory infiltrates and the hemangioendothelioma (as in the cases discussed above) alone would probably not account for sudden death, but could have played a triggering role. Our cases are consistent with the triple-risk model of SIDS, a hypothesis consisting of underlying biological vulnerability to exogenous stressors or triggering factors in a critical developmental period [59]. Further studies on triggering factors and related mechanisms will lead to a better understanding of complex interactions involved in the pathophysiology of SIDS. The cases presented here seem to usefully contribute to the orientation of research in this field [160, 214, 273].

IV.2.6 Paraganglia Hyperplasia

Paraganglia hyperplasia was detected in 25% of our SIDS infants and resulted in prolonged hypoxia. Our experience suggests that this abnormality is not so marked in intercarotid as in mediastinal glomera. In fact, the mediastinal glomera are a part of the cardiac nerve plexus and are functionally more pertinent to the cardiocirculatory regulation [169, 184, 222, 223]. Enlargement of the aorticopulmonary paraganglia (APP) in infants dying of SIDS was confirmed in our infants by the use of sophisticated morphometric techniques. Hyperplasia of the APP can be readily observed from sections under the low power objective of the microscope, but an unequivocal proof of glomic cell proliferation can only be confirmed by morphometric measurement [222].

Previous reports describe a more extensive and prominent distribution of paraganglia cells in human fetuses and infants than in adults [81]. Our results confirm this aspect: the APP of control infants were greater in number and size at birth and decreased dramatically during the first year of life. The mechanism underlying this morphological variation is not yet known. Programmed cell death may play a role in the process [81, 222]. In some SIDS victims an underlying vulnerability may be a reduction in the volume of the ARCn [58, 163], which is considered an essential chemoreceptive component of the neuroanatomic circuitry involved in cardiorespiratory modulation [286]. The interactions of the ARCn with the peripheral chemoreceptors have been investigated [222]. The paraganglia hyperplasia observed in some SIDS infants could be compensatory, beginning from alterations in the central chemoreceptor mechanisms [222, 224].

IV.2.7 Long QT Syndrome

A notable example of multifocal apoptotic degeneration of the sinus node occurs in victims dying of the LQT syndrome, a clinical entity characterized by sinus bradycardia [96, 105, 210]. Sudden unexpected death is one of the clinical characteristics of the LQT syndrome and has often been found to be mediated by lethal ventricular arrhythmias. It is logical to anticipate that the normal occurrence of apoptotic cell death during postnatal morphogenesis of the sinus node will periodically distort or suppress normal sinus rhythm [106]. Moreover, in the LQT syndrome apoptotic destruction involves not only the myocytes of the sinus node but also many local nerves and ganglia [96, 105].

QT prolongation could be dangerous in babies and a possible cause of their fatal arrhythmia [76, 260], but solid evidence of its occurrence is still lacking and such an association is still a matter of controversy. The capricious nature of episodic QT prolongation documented in human infants poses difficulties in demonstrating lethal cardiac electrical instability [96, 210].

Schwartz et al. [254], in a 19-year prospective study, performed follow-up electrocardiography in an unselected population of over 33,000 infants, and concluded that congenital prolongation of the QT interval accounts for a proportion of SIDS cases. Their results underline the potential value of neonatal electrocardiographic screening for an early identification of a prolonged long QT interval and consequent preventive treatment of the affected infants [221, 254]. However, Schwartz et al. admitted that the LQT syndrome may account for only a fraction of the crib death cases, and precise quantification of this fraction remains difficult despite the data obtained from their large epidemiological study [254, 255]. Guntheroth and Spiers [76] state that submitting all infants and newborns to electrocardiographic screening would be ineffective and a waste of medical resources, and it would cruelly alarm thousands of parents.

Recent studies also indicate further close clinicopathogenetic analogies with arrhythmogenic lethal late repolarization, attended by fetal developmental impairments of the conduction system, often resulting in accessory AV pathways, whose high frequency in SIDS has been documented in the present cases and is entirely consistent with junctional tachycardia [247]. An important report, in this connection, is that of Kuo et al. [126] who emphasize the possible role of the conduction system among the ontogenetic substrates of the Ito abnormalities. This genetic clinicopathological suggestion is further substantiated by recent work coauthored by Rossi [16] on the life-threatening potential of WPW syndrome, whose common accessory AV pathway substrate was proven occasionally to have a genetic association [67].

Viskin et al. [276] recommend genetic screening in every case of probable LQT syndrome, and state that a positive result will confirm the diagnosis but that no mutations are found in many patients with a definite diagnosis of LQT syndrome, so a negative result is not very helpful. In any case, genetic testing might take months, and the patient needs treatment [210, 276].

Concluding Remarks

V

Never again will there be in it an infant who lives but a few days, or an old man who does not live out his years; he who dies at a hundred will be thought a mere youth; he who fails to reach a hundred will be considered accursed. (Isaiah 65:20)

Crib death or SIDS is defined as the sudden death of an infant which is unexpected from the history and not explained by post-mortem examination or review of the death scene [280]. Despite a wide spectrum of proposed theories, its etiology remains uncertain.

SIUD (sudden intrauterine unexplained death) is late fetal death before the complete expulsion or removal of the fetus from the mother [115]. Advances in maternal and fetal care have produced a significant reduction in perinatal mortality, but have not significantly changed the prevalence of SIUD. SIUD represents about one-half of perinatal mortalities, with a prevalence of 5–12 per 1,000 births [1, 253].

Knowledge of the ante- and post-mortem aspects of SIDS and SIUD is of international public concern, since its prevention would save a great number of potentially productive citizens. However, the classification criteria for SIDS and late fetal unexplained death, the criteria for study and the methods of post-mortem examination are still too multifaceted and controversial. Nevertheless, in recent years, further progress in the diagnostic and scientific–instrumental procedures in SIDS and stillbirth ("the last diagnosis") have opened to the anatomic and forensic pathologist important new avenues for research in this area.

In order to obtain a correct epicritic diagnosis, anatomic and forensic pathologists are required to analyze, in as complete a way as possible, all morphological aspects of each SIDS as well as SIUD case. It is necessary that the pathologist applies new tools and methodologies of investigation to each case and acquires a deepening knowledge in order to be able to interpret those signs that may be considered significant.

The observation of frequent anomalies, mostly congenital, of the autonomic nervous system structures in both SIDS [133, 163, 174] and SIUD [167, 171, 174] indicates a continuity between these two pathologies. Our research upholds a new approach to SIDS which involves the recognition of its analogical link with SIUD. Indeed, early SIDS may well depend upon postnatal block of respiratory reflexes for fetal survival, involving the Kölliker-Fuse nucleus, or upon impaired development of central circuitry for respiratory reflexogenesis [79]. The acronym SIUD-SIDS underlines a possible common morphological substrate.

Despite the nonspecificity of most of the cardiac conduction findings in SIDS, it is believed that they, in association with altered neurovegetative stimuli [163, 254], could underlie potentially malignant arrhythmias, providing morphological support for the cardiac concept of crib death [210]. In fact, the coincidence of other events (such as fever, vomiting or diarrhea and electrolytic imbalance) and active cell death in the conduction system seems to be crucial in causing crib death, whereas cell death and otherwise innocuous events are harmless if they occur separately. It is therefore important that we recognize and act upon as many of these contributing causes, including sleeping position, as possible.

Respiratory derangements in infants appear to be predominantly neurogenic in nature since our observations indicate that such derangements can mainly be ascribed to prenatal and/or congenital developmental abnormalities compromising the reflexogenic neuroreceptors, whether central or peripheral. Their anatomical location and their particular functional effects are likely to interfere with the rhythmic and biochemical modulation of breathing and heartbeat. But what makes the problem more complicated is the very dichotomous difference in reflexogenic physiology. This dichotomy may even became life-threatening during the pre- and postpartum periods. This may account for the fact that the problem of SIDS is still a perplexing and incompletely understood dilemma, and this has motivated our anatomopathological team to pursue coordinated investigations into the crib death infant side by side with the unexpected stillborn fetus in late pregnancy, such deaths being intimately related to the pathological/anatomical/physiological problem of vital oxygen supply before and after birth [171]. As the exact mechanism of cardiopulmonary failure in SIDS and SIUD is still unknown, all autonomic related central nervous system regions and neurotransmitters are open to further investigation.

It is not up to the pathologist to draw conclusions about the clinical diagnosis and prevention of SIDS. Even though the pathologist is always involved too late to avoid the tragedy, he/she yet can underline the need for a thorough post-mortem examination of every SIDS victim.

The search will be continued in the infant and fetal cardiac conduction and autonomic nervous systems. To supplement the clinicophysiological findings in infants and term fetuses dying suddenly and unexpectedly, a deeper insight is needed from microscopic research (histology, ultrastructure, immunohistochemistry), the extreme specialization of which requires centers with the necessary expertise [174, 210].

The necessary cardiac and neuropathological studies seeking to identify the morphological substrate in crib death requires the examination of a large number of cases using homogeneous and standardized criteria. A complete examination of the cardiac conduction and nervous systems in serial sections allows an objective dimensional and architectural evaluation of all the inherent pertinent anatomic areas [174, 210, 214]. This requires many sections and the systematic application of appropriate histological techniques (e.g. H&E, Klüver-Barrera, and trichromic Heidenhain stains), histochemical techniques (e.g. Glees-Marsland for neurons and neurofibrils, Bielschowsky for axons and dendrites, Mallory's PTAH for glia), and immunohistochemical techniques (to study apoptosis, various neuroreceptor structures, the expression of specific genes, etc.). Moreover, such complete examination of the cardiac conduction system requires the availability of properly trained histotechnicians. It should also be underlined that, due to the architectural variability of the conduction system and brainstem, wrong indications on the involved structures and extension can result from the examination of single and casually chosen sections [174, 210]. I am therefore convinced that the autopsy protocol for SIDS victims, as already internationally approved [30, 125], should always include examination of the cardiac conduction and central, peripheral and autonomic nervous systems according to the guidelines described in this work and available on the web site of the Institute of Pathology, University of Milan (http://users.unimi.it/~pathol/pathol_e.html).

Summary

SIDS, or crib death, is defined as the sudden death of an infant under 1 year of age which remains unexplained after a thorough investigation of the case, including the performance of a complete autopsy, examination of the death scene, and a review of the clinical history. SIDS is the most frequent death-causing syndrome occurring during the first year of life, striking one baby in every 700–1,000. Since it is a particularly tragic event for a healthy vigorous infant to die suddenly and unexpectedly, it is not surprising that the subject is of great medical and public interest.

There is an association between SIDS and sleep, and this is combined with data indicating impaired autonomic function in infants who subsequently die of SIDS or suffer apparent life-threatening events (ALTE). The pathology of SIDS is included in the extended domain of neonatal pathology, particularly if within the diagnosis of SIDS one wishes to include so-called "borderline" SIDS not definitely separable from the unifying concept of the syndrome.

SIUD (sudden intrauterine unexplained death) is late fetal death before the complete expulsion or removal of the fetus from the mother. Advances in maternal and fetal care have produced a significant reduction in perinatal mortality, but have not changed the prevalence of SIUD. SIUD represents about one-half of perinatal mortalities, with a prevalence of 5–12 per 1,000 births, and its etiology is largely unexplained.

Knowledge of the ante- and post-mortem aspects of SIDS and SIUD is of international public concern, since its prevention would save a great number of potentially productive citizens.

In the anatomic/pathological concept, different findings have been reported as possible SIDS substrates: brainstem abnormalities, cardiac conduction system developmental defects, immaturity of the paraganglia, and hyper- or hypoplasia of the carotid bodies. Overall, the abnormalities of the autonomic nervous and cardiac conduction systems do represent a plausible basis for SIDS being reflexogenic in nature (dive, feigned death, cardio-auditory reflexes, Ondine syndrome). Vagal cardiorespiratory reflexes, if pathological, could lead to SIDS.

From 1987 to 2003, at the Institute of Pathology, University of Milan, many cases of sudden infant and fetal death have been analyzed, since the Institute is the referral center for SIDS and late unexplained fetal death for the Lombardy Region (DGR no. 11693 of 20/6/2002). Italian Law no. 31 of 2 February 2006 "Regulations for Diagnostic Post Mortem Investigation in Victims of Sudden Infant Death Syndrome (SIDS) and unexpected fetal death" designates the Institute of Pathology of the University of Milan as the national referral center being a recognized institution competent in this issue. From an even larger number of cases, a total of 120 SIDS victims, 37 infant controls and 60 late fetal stillbirths, after the exclusion of violent causes, were selected for this work.

For each analyzed case, the cardiac conduction system was removed in two blocks for paraffin embedding: block 1 (the sinoatrial node, SAN) and block 2 (the atrioventricular, AV, system). The brainstem was divided into three blocks according to a simplified procedure for brainstem examination, requiring a much lower number of sections and less work for the histotechnicians. For each brainstem nucleus (in particular, the arcuate nucleus (ARCn) and parabrachial/Kölliker-Fuse complex), using serial sections stained with Klüver-Barrera stain, the neuronal cell body areas, neuronal density, transverse section areas and volume were evaluated. The statistical significance of the differences between the means of the two fetus groups (SIUD and stillbirth controls) and two infant groups (SIDS and infant controls) was determined by one-way analysis of variance. The carotid bifurcations, cardiac plexus ganglia and paraganglia were embedded separately and serially sectioned. In selected cases, immunohistochemistry studies were performed on sections of the cardiac conduction system, brainstem, and coronary arteries.

The SIDS victims did not show any abnormality of the ordinary myocardium, while the core of the heart, where cardiac rhythm arises and spreads, showed some abnormalities. More than one cardiac conduction change was present in the same infant, but no peculiar cardiac combined anomaly was observed. Areas of resorptive degeneration were detected in 97% of SIDS infants and in 75% of controls. Macrophages were sometimes present adjacent to the small foci of degeneration, acting eventually as scavenger cells.

The developmental abnormalities in SIDS include long dendritic spines, markers of neuronal immaturity, and hypoplasia of the brainstem nuclei. In SIDS mono- or bilateral hypoplasia or even agenesis of the ARCn is particularly frequent. It was observed and morphometrically studied in 56.06% of our SIDS infants, and was found to be bilateral in 17.9% and monolateral (always the right side) in 12.16%. We further considered the shape of the cell body, nucleus and nucleolus.

Comparative analysis of serial histological sections obtained from the pons and mesencephalon of SIUD and SIDS victims and those of the two control groups made it possible to define the morphological features of the three principal nuclei of the human PB/KF complex: the lateral parabrachial (lPB) nucleus, the medial parabrachial (mPB) nucleus, and the Kölliker-Fuse (KF) nucleus.

A combined morphological post-mortem study of the cardiac conduction system and brainstem was performed in 42 SIDS infants and in 12 controls. Mahaim fibers were observed in 16% of control and in 17% of SIDS infants with the ARCn histologically well developed, and in 50% (severe bilateral hypoplasia) to 71% (monolateral hypoplasia) of SIDS infants with ARCn hypoplasia. The Mahaim fibers were significantly more frequent in SIDS infants with ARCn hypoplasia than in those with a well-developed ARCn (control and other SIDS infants; p<0.005).

Hyperplasia of the aorticopulmonary paraganglia was detected in 25% of SIDS victims. The cell clusters and cell diameters were not significantly different from those of age-matched controls. Two SIDS infants showed intracapsular glomus in the left stellate ganglion and five SIDS infants showed inflammatory foci in the right stellate ganglion.

The observation of frequent anomalies, mostly congenital, of the autonomic nervous system structures, both in SIDS and in SIUD indicates a continuity between these two pathologies. Our research supports a new approach to SIDS which involves the recognition of its analogical link with SIUD. Indeed, early SIDS may well depend upon postnatal block of respiratory reflexes for fetal survival, involving the KF nucleus, or upon impaired development of central circuitry for respiratory reflexogenesis. The acronym SIUD-SIDS underlines possible common morphological substrata.

The search will be continued for a better understanding of what is normal and what is abnormal in the infant and fetal cardiac conduction and nervous systems and the herein presented histopathological findings seems to usefully contribute literature information for crib death as well as for unexplained perinatal death.

References

1. Ahlenius I, Thomassen P (1999) The changing panorama of late fetal death in Sweden between 1984 and 1991. Acta Obstet Gynecol Scand 78:408–414
2. Alfonsi G, Crippa M (1994) Tecniche istologiche e immunoistochimiche di seriatura e colorazione del sistema di conduzione e nervoso cardiaco. Pathologica 86:444–449
3. Anderson KR, Hill RW (1982) Occlusive lesions of cardiac conducting tissue arteries in sudden infant death syndrome. Pediatrics 69:50–52
4. Anderson RH (2000) Sudden and unexpected death in infancy and the conduction system of the heart. Cardiovasc Pathol 9:147–148
5. Anderson RH, Bouton J, Burrow CT, Smith A (1974) Sudden death in infancy: a study of cardiac specialized tissue. Br Med J 2:135–139
6. Anderson WAD, Dmytryk ET (1946) Primary tumor of the heart containing epithelium-like elements. Am J Pathol 22:337–343
7. Anderson WR, Edland JF, Schenk EA (1970) Conducting system changes in the sudden infant death syndrome. Am J Pathol 59:35a
8. Arbustini E, Diegoli M, Grasso M, Fasani R, D'Armini A, Martinelli L, Goggi C, Campana C, Gavazzi A, Vigano M (1993) Expression of proliferating cell markers in normal and diseased human hearts. Am J Cardiol 72:608–614
9. Arntzen A, Moum T, Magnum P, Bakketeig LS (1995) Is the higher postneonatal mortality in lower social status due to SIDS? Acta Paediatr 84:188–192
10. Askenazi SS, Perlman M (1979) Pulmonary hypoplasia: lung weight and radial alveolar count as criteria of diagnosis. Arch Dis Child 54:614–618
11. Atkinson JB, Virmani R (1991) The endomyocardial biopsy: techniques, indications and limitations. In: Virmani R, Atkinson JB, Fenoglio J (eds) Cardiovascular pathology. Saunders, Philadelphia, p 210
12. Balk SJ, Bearer CF, Etzel RA, Falk H, Hendrick JG, Miller MD, Miller RW, Rogan W, She KM, Simon PR (1997) Environmental tobacco smoke: a hazard to children (RE9716). Pediatrics 99:639–642
13. Bancroft J, Stevens A (1982) Theory and practice of histological techniques, 2nd edn. Churchill Livingstone, New York
14. Baracchini A, Rossomando V, Chiaravallotti G, Buti G, Ceccarelli M (1995) Apparent life threatening events (ALTE): prelude to SIDS? Minerva Pediatr 47:393–399
15. Barton JR, Boheler KR, Brand NJ, Thomas PS (1995) Molecular biology of cardiac development and growth. Springer-Verlag, Berlin Heidelberg New York
16. Basso C, Corrado D, Rossi L, Thiene G (2001) Ventricular preexcitation in children and young adults: atrial myocarditis as a possible trigger of sudden death. Circulation 103:269–275
17. Benedetti G (1994) Risvolti giuridico-pratici della morte improvvisa cardiaca che attengono alla Procura della Repubblica. Pathologica 86:430–433
18. Berry PJ (1992) Pathological findings in SIDS. J Clin Pathol 45 [11 Suppl]:11–16
19. Bharati S, Lev M (1986) Congenital abnormalities in the conduction system in sudden death in young adults. J Am Coll Cardiol 8:1096–1104
20. Bharati S, Lev M (1994) Conduction system findings in sudden death in young adults with a history of bronchial asthma. J Am Coll Cardiol 23:741–746

21. Bharati S, Dreifus L, Bucheleres G, Molthan M, Covitz W, Isenberg HS, Lev M (1985) The conduction system in patients with a prolonged QT interval. J Am Coll Cardiol 6:1110–1119

22. Bharati S, Krongrad E, Lev M (1985) Study of the conduction system in a population of patients with sudden infant death syndrome. Pediatr Cardiol 6:29–40

23. Bigger HR, Silvestri JM, Shott S, Weese Mayer DE (1998) Influence of increased survival in very low birth weight, low weight, and normal birth weight infants on the incidence of sudden infant death syndrome in the United States: 1985–1991. J Pediatr 133:73–78

24. Bolande RP, Leistikow EA, Wartman F, Louis T (1996) The development of preatherosclerotic coronary artery lesions in perinatal piglets. Biol Neonate 69:109–118

25. Bouchardy B, Majno G (1974) Histopathology of early infarcts. Am J Pathol 74:301–330

26. Boyle FM, Vance JC, Najman JM, Thearle MJ (1996) The mental health impact of stillbirth, neonatal death or SIDS: prevalence and patterns of distress among mothers. Soc Sci Med 43:1273–1282

27. Brooks JG, Kattwinkel J, Keenan ME, Malloy M, Scheers NJ, Willinger M (2000) Changing concepts of sudden infant death syndrome: implications for infant sleeping environment and sleep position. Pediatrics 105:650–656

28. Buja GF, Corrado D, Pellegrino PA, Nava A, Thiene G (1986) Fatal paroxysmal supraventricular tachycardia in an infant. Chest 90:145–146

29. Burchell A, Lyall H, Busuttil A, Bell E, Hume R (1992) Glucose metabolism and hypoglycemia in SIDS. J Clin Pathol 45 [11 Suppl]:39–45

30. Byard RW, Krous HF (2001) Sudden infant death syndrome. Problems, progress and possibilities. Arnold, Hodder Headline Group, London

31. Calderoli R, Martini F, Galli S, Matturri L (2002) Post mortem discipline on the sudden infant death syndrome (SIDS) and of unexpected late fetal stillbirth victims. In: Proceedings of the 7th SIDS International Conference, Florence, Italy, p 135

32. Campbel MJ, Julious SA, Peterson CK, Tobias A (2001) Atmospheric pressure and sudden infant death syndrome in Cook County, Chicago. Paediatr Perinatal Epidemiol 3:287–289

33. Carroll-Pankhurst C, Mortimer EA (2001) Sudden infant death syndrome, bedsharing, parental weight, and age at death. Pediatrics 107:530–536

34. Castano P, Cocco L, De Barbieri A, D'Este L, Floriani F, Gheri G, Mondello MR, Papa S, Petriglieri P, Pizzini G, Ridola C, Sirigu P, Spinella S (1986) Anatomia Umana. Edi-Ermes, Milan, pp 434–440

35. Centers for Disease Control and Prevention (CDC) (1996) Sudden infant death syndrome – United States, 1983–1994. MMWR Morb Mortal Wkly Rep 45:859–863

36. Chamberlin NL, Saper CB (1994) Topographic organization of respiratory responses to glutamate microstimulation of the parabrachial nucleus in the rat. J Neurosci 414:6500–6510

37. Cohle SD, Lie JT (1991) Pathologic changes of the cardiac conduction tissue in sudden unexpected death. A review. Pathol Annu 26 Pt 2:33–57

38. Colombo B, Ottaviani G, Ramos SG, Matturri L (1998) Apoptosis in cardiac conduction system in sudden infant death syndrome (SIDS): preliminary results. In: Proceedings of the 5th SIDS International Conference, Rouen, France, p 157

39. Cooper RM, Lumley J (1996) Mother's knowledge of the risk factors and anxiety about SIDS. J Paediatr Child Health 32:310–315

40. Corr CA, Fuller H, Barnickol CA, Corr DM (eds) (1991) Sudden infant death syndrome: who can help and how. Springer, New York

41. Côtè A, Hum C, Brouillette RT, Themens M (1998) Frequency and timing of recurrent events in infants using home cardiorespiratory monitors. J Pediatr 132:783–789

42. Cotzias CS, Paterson-Brown S, Fisk NM (1999) Prospective risk of unexplained stillbirth in singleton pregnancies at term: population based analysis. BMJ 319:287–288

43. Crippa M, Alfonsi G (1991) Tecniche di studio del sistema di conduzione cardiaco. BIO-Informazioni, BIO-OPTICA, Milan, pp 55–58

44. Cummings MC, Winterford CM, Walker NI (1997) Apoptosis. Am J Surg Pathol 21:88–101

45. Davies MJ, Anderson RH, Becker AE (1983) The conduction system of the heart. Butterworth, London

46. Dawes GS, Fox HE, Leduc BM, Liggins GC, Richards RT (1972) Respiratory movements and rapid eye movement sleep in the fetal lamb. J Physiol 220:119–143

47. de Sa DJ (1978) Stress response and its relationship to cystic (pseudofollicular) change in the definitive cortex of the adrenal gland in stillborn infants. Arch Dis Child 53:769–776

48. Doerr W (1957) Die morphologie des reizleitungssystemes ihre orthologie und pathologie. In: Spang K (ed) Rhythmusstörungen des herzens. Thieme, Stuttgart, pp 11–16

49. Doerr W, Schiebler TH (1963) Pathologische anatomie des reizleitungssystems. In: Bargmann W, Doerr W (eds) Das Herz des Menschen. Thieme, Stuttgart

50. Dony C, Gruss P (1987) Proto-oncogene c-fos expression in growth regions of fetal bone and mesodermal tissue. Nature 299:711–714

51. Eisenberg MS, Mengert TJ (2000) Cardiac resuscitation. N Engl J Med 343:1206–1209

52. Emery JL (1993) Child abuse, sudden infant death syndrome, and unexpected infant death. Am J Dis Child 147:1097–1100

53. Eyzaguirre C, Nishi K, Fidone S (1972) Chemoreceptor synapses in the carotid body. Fed Proc 31:1385–1393

54. Fares T, McCulloch KM, Raju TN (1997) Intrauterine cocaine exposure and the risk for sudden infant death syndrome: a meta-analysis. J Perinatol 17:179–182

55. Ferris JA (1972) Cot death – why not the heart? Med Sci Law 12:173–177

56. Ferris JA (1973) Hypoxic changes in conducting tissue of the heart in sudden death in infancy syndrome. Br Med J 2:23–25

57. Ferris JA, Aherne WA (1971) Cartilage in relation to the conducting tissue of the heart in sudden death. Lancet 1:64–66

58. Filiano JJ, Kinney HC (1992) Arcuate nucleus hypoplasia in the sudden infant death syndrome. J Neuropathol Exp Neurol 51:394–403

59. Filiano JJ, Kinney HC (1994) A perspective on neuropathologic findings in victims of sudden infant death syndrome: the triple risk model. Biol Neonate 65:194–197

60. Fleming KA (1992) Viral respiratory infection and SIDS. J Clin Pathol 45 [11 Suppl]:29–32

61. Frahna JG, Pollack HA (2001) A competing risk model of sudden infant death syndrome incidents in two US birth cohorts. J Pediatr 138:661–667

62. Freeman DH, Malloy MH (2000) Birth weight- and gestational age-specific sudden infant death syndrome mortality: United States, 1991 versus 1995. Pediatrics 105:1227–1231

63. Gerbitz KD, Jaksch M (1994) Mitochondrial DNA, aging and sudden infant death syndrome. Eur J Clin Chem Clin Biochem 32:487–488

64. Gerlis LM (1996) Covert congenital cardiovascular malformations discovered in an autopsy series of nearly 5000 cases. Cardiovasc Pathol 5:11–19

65. Ghidoni P, Giudici E, Matturri L, Rossi L (1986) Extranodal specialized sinoatrial cells. Anal Quant Cytol Histol 8:255–258

66. Gilbert-Barness E (1997) Potter's pathology of the fetus and infant. Mosby Year Book, St Louis

67. Gollob MH, Green MS, Tang A S-L, Gollob T, Karibe A, Hassa A, Ahmad F, Lozado R, Shah G, Fananapazir L, Bachinski L, Roberts R (2001) Identification of a gene responsible for familial Wolff-Parkinson-White syndrome. N Engl J Med 344:1823–1831

68. Gordon AE, Saadi AT, MacKenzie DA, James VS, Elton RA, Veir DM, Busuttil A, Blackwell CC (1999) The protective effect of breast feeding in relation to sudden infant death syndrome (SIDS): II. The effect of human milk and infant formula preparations on binding Clostridium perfringens to epithelial cells. FEMS Immunol Med Microbiol 25:167–173

69. Grant RP (1962) The embryology of ventricular flow pathways in man. Circulation 25:756–779

70. Green A (1993) Biochemical screening in newborn siblings of cases of SIDS. Arch Dis Child 68:793–796

71. Gregersen N, Winter V, Jensen PK, Holmskov A, Kolvraa S, Andresen BS, Christensen E, Bross P, Lundemose JB, Gregersen M (1995) Prenatal diagnosis of medium-chain acyl-CoA dehydrogenase (MCAD) deficiency in a family with a previous fatal case of sudden unexpected death in childhood. Prenat Diagn 15:82–86

72. Guareschi M, Ottaviani G, Ramos SG, Matturri L (1998) Morte improvvisa del lattante (SIDS): un caso con vie accessorie e resorptive degeneration. Pathologica 90:294–297

73. Guntheroth WG (1995) Crib death: the sudden infant death syndrome, 3rd edn. Futura, Mount Kisko, New York

74. Guntheroth WG (1999) Risk factors for SIDS. In: Proceedings of the 19th International Symposium on Neonatal Intensive Care, Milan, Italy, p 36

75. Guntheroth WG, Spiers PS (1992) Sleeping prone and the risk of sudden infant death syndrome. JAMA 267:2359–2362

76. Guntheroth WG, Spiers PS (1996) Are bedding and rebreathing suffocation a cause of SIDS? Pediatr Pulmonol 22:335–341

77. Guntheroth WG, Spiers PS (1999) Prolongation of the QT interval and the sudden infant death syndrome. Pediatrics 10:813–814

78. Guntheroth WG, Spiers PS (2001) Thermal stress in sudden infant death: is there an ambiguity with the rebreathing hypothesis? Pediatrics 107:693–698

79. Guntheroth WG, Spiers PS (2002) The triple risk hypotheses in sudden infant death syndrome. Pediatrics 110:E64

80. Haas JE, Taylor JA, Bergman AB, Van Belle G, Felgenhauer JL, Siebert JR, Benjamin DR (1993) Relationship between epidemiologic risk factors and clinicopathologic findings in the sudden infant death syndrome. Pediatrics 91:106–112

81. Hervonen A, Vaalasti A, Partanen M, Kanerva L, Vaalasti T (1976) The paraganglia, a persisting endocrine system in man. Am J Anat 146:207–210

82. Hirano T, Simbulan D, Kumayawa T (1994) Effects of kainic acid in the parabrachial region for ongoing respiratory activity and reflexive respiratory suppression. Brain Res 665:54–62

83. Ho SY, Anderson RH (1988) Conduction tissue and SIDS. Ann N Y Acad Sci 533:176–190

84. Ho SY, Mortimer G, Anderson RH, Pomerance A, Keelings JW (1985) Conduction system defects in three perinatal patients with arrhythmia. Br Heart J 53:158–163

85. Hockenbery D (1995) Defining apoptosis. Am J Pathol 146:16–18

86. Hoffman HJ, Damus K, Hillman L, Kangrad E (1988) Risk factors for SIDS. Results of the National Institute of Child Health and Human Development SIDS cooperation epidemiological study. Ann N Y Acad Sci 533:13–30

87. James TN (1968) Sudden death in babies: new observation in the heart. Am J Cardiol 22:479–506

88. James TN (1970) Cardiac conduction system: fetal and postnatal development. Am J Cardiol 25:213–226

89. James TN (1976) Sudden death of babies. Circulation 53:1–2

90. James TN (1983) Change and sudden death. J Am Coll Cardiol 1:164–183

91. James TN (1983) The Mikamo lecture. Structure and function of AV junction. Jpn Circ J 47:1–47

92. James TN (1985) Crib death. J Am Coll Cardiol 5:1185–1187

93. James TN (1985) Normal variations and pathologic changes in structure of the cardiac conduction system and their functional significance. J Am Coll Cardiol 5:71B–78B

94. James TN (1993) Congenital disorders of cardiac rhythm and conduction. J Cardiovasc Electrophysiol 4:702–718

95. James TN (1994) Normal and abnormal consequences of apoptosis in the human heart. From postnatal morphogenesis to paroxysmal arrhythmias. Circulation 90:556–573

96. James TN (1996) Long reflections on the QT interval: the sixth annual Gordon K. Moe lecture. J Cardiovasc Electrophysiol 7:738–759

97. James TN (1997) Apoptosis in congenital heart disease. Coron Artery Dis 8:599–616

98. James TN (1998) Normal and abnormal consequences of apoptosis in the human heart. Annu Rev Physiol 60:309–325

99. James TN (1999) Apoptosis in cardiac disease. Am J Med 107:606–620

100. James TN (2001) The internodal pathways of the human heart. Prog Cardiovasc Dis 43:495–535

101. James TN (2002) Structure and function of the sinus node, AV node and His bundle of the human heart: Part I – stucture. Prog Cardiovasc Dis 45:235–267

102. James TN (2003) Structure and function of the sinus node, AV node and His bundle of the human heart: Part II – function. Prog Cardiovasc Dis 45:327–360

103. James TN, Marshall TK (1976) De Subitaneis Mortibus XVIII. Persistent fetal dispersion of the atrioventricular node and His bundle within the central fibrous body. Circulation 6:1026–1034

104. James TN, Froggatt P, Marshall TK (1967) Sudden death in young athletes. Ann Intern Med 67:1013–1021

105. James TN, Froggatt P, Atkinson WJ Jr, Lurie PR, McNamara DG, Miller WW, Schloss GT, Carroll JF, North RL (1978) De subitaneis mortibus XXX. Observations on the pathophysiology of the QT syndromes with special reference to the neuropathology of the heart. Circulation 57:1221–1231

106. James TN, Nichols MM, Sapire DW, Di Patre PL, Lopez SM (1996) Complete heart block and fatal right ventricular failure in an infant. Circulation 93:1588–1600

107. James TN, St. Martin E, Willis PW 3rd, Lohr TO (1996) Apoptosis as a possible cause of gradual development of complete heart block and fatal arrhythmias associated with absence of the AV node, sinus node and internodal pathways. Circulation 93:1424–1438

108. Jankus A (1976) The cardiac conduction system in sudden infant death syndrome: a report on three cases. Pathology 8:275–280

109. Jeffery HE, Page M, Post EJ, Wood AK (1995) Physiological studies of gastro-oesophageal reflux and airway protective responses in young animal and human infant. Clin Exp Pharmacol Physiol 22:544–549

110. Jeffery HE, Megevan A, Page M (1999) Why the prone position is a risk factor for sudden infant death syndrome. Pediatrics 104:263–269

111. Jenkins RO, Craig PJ, Goessler W, Irgolic KJ (1998) Antimony leaching from cot mattresses and sudden infant death syndrome (SIDS). Hum Exp Toxicol 17:138–139

112. Kaada B (1986) Sudden infant death syndrome: the possible role of "the fear paralysis reflex". Norwegian University Press, Oslo

113. Kahn A, Blum D, Muller MF, Montauk L, Bochner A, Monod N, Plouin P, Samson-Dollfus D, Delagree EH (1986) Sudden infant death syndrome in twins: a comparison of sibling histories. Pediatrics 78:146–150

114. Kajstura J, Mansukhani M, Cheng W, Reiss K, Krajewski S, Reed JC, Quaini F, Sonnenblick EH, Anversa P (1995) Programmed cell death and expression of the protooncogene bcl-2 in myocytes during postnatal maturation of the heart. Exp Cell Res 219:110–121

115. Kalousek DK, Gilbert-Barness E (1997) Causes of stillbirth and neonatal death. In: Potter's pathology of the fetus and infant. Mosby-Year book, New York, pp 128–162

116. Keith A, Flack MW (1906) The auricolo-ventricular bundle of the human heart. Lancet 2:359–364

117. Kelmanson IA (1994) Relationship between the incidence of sudden infant death syndrome (SIDS) and other causes of infant mortality in the industrialized countries. Paediatr Perinatol Epidemiol 8:166–172

118. Kinney HC, Filiano JJ, Harper RM (1992) The neuropathology of the sudden infant death syndrome. A review. J Neuropathol Exp Neurol 51:115–126

119. Kinney HC, O'Donnel TJ, Kriger P, White WF (1993) Early developmental changes in H3-nicotine binding in the human brainstem. Neuroscience 55:1127–1138

120. Kinney HC, Filiano JJ, Panigraphy A, Rava LA, White WF (1995) Anatomic and neurochemical studies of the ventral medulla oblongata in early life. Observation relevant to the sudden infant death syndrome. In: Trouth CO, Millis RH, Kiwull-Schone H, Schlafke ME (eds) Ventral brainstem mechanisms and control respiration and blood pressure. Dekker, New York, pp 589–609

121. Kinney HC, Filiano JJ, Sleeper LA, Mandell F, Valdes-Dapena M, White WF (1995) Decreased muscarinic receptor binding in the arcuate nucleus in sudden infant death syndrome. Science

269:1446–1450

122. Klonoff-Cohen HS, Edelstein SL, Lefkowitz ES, Srinivasan IP, Kaegi D, Chang JC, Wiley KJ (1995) The effect of passive smoking and tobacco exposure through breast milk on sudden infant death syndrome. JAMA 273:795–798

123. Knobel HH, Chen CJ, Liang KY (1995) Sudden infant death syndrome in relation to weather and optimetrically measured air pollution in Taiwan. Pediatrics 96:1106–1110

124. Kozakewich HPW, McManus BM, Vawter G (1982) The sinus node in sudden infant death syndrome. Circulation 65:1242–1246

125. Krous H (1996) Instruction and reference manual for the International standardized autopsy protocol for sudden unexpected infant death. J SIDS Infant Mortality 1:203–246

126. Kuo HC, Cheng CF, Clark RB, Lin JJ, Lin JL, Gu Y, Ikeda Y, Chu PH, Ross J Jr, Giles WR, Chien KR (2001) A defect in the Kv channel-interacting protein 2 (KchIP2) gene leads to a complete loss of Ito and confers susceptibility to ventricular tachycardia. Cell 107:801–812

127. Lack EE (1994) Pathology of adrenal and extra-adrenal paraganglia. W.B. Saunders, Philadelphia

128. Lanting CI, Boersma ER (1996) Lipid in infant nutrition and their impact on later development. Curr Opin Lipidol 7:43–47

129. Lavezzi AM, Matturri L, Ballabio G, Ottaviani G, Rossi L (2002) Study of the cytoarchitecture of the parabrachial/Kölliker-Fuse complex in SIDS and fetal late stillbirth. In: Proceedings of the 7th International Conference on SIDS, Florence, Italy, p 132

130. Lavezzi AM, Ottaviani G, De Ruberto F, Fichera G, Matturri L (2002) Prognostic significance of different biomarkers (DNA content, PCNA, karyotype) in colorectal adenomas. Anticancer Res 22:2077–2082

131. Lavezzi AM, Ottaviani G, Matturri L (2003) Identification of neurons responding to hypoxia in sudden infant death syndrome (SIDS). Pathol Int 53:769–774

132. Lavezzi AM, Ottaviani G, Ballabio G, Rossi L, Matturri L (2004) Preliminary study on the cytoarchitecture of the human parabrachial/Kölliker-Fuse complex, with reference to sudden infant death syndrome and sudden intrauterine unexplained death. Pediatr Dev Pathol 7:171–179

133. Lavezzi AM, Ottaviani G, Mauri M, Matturri L (2004) Hypoplasia of the arcuate nucleus and maternal smoking during pregnancy, in perinatal and infant sudden unexpected death. Neuropathology 24:284–289

134. Lavezzi AM, Ottaviani G, Matturri L (2004) Involvement of somatostatin in breathing control before and after birth, and in perinatal and infant sudden unexplained death. Folia Neuropathol 42:59–65

135. Lavezzi AM, Ottaviani G, Matturri L (2004) Role of somatostatin and apoptosis in breathing control in sudden perinatal and infant unexplained death. Clin Neuropathol 23:304–310

136. Lavezzi AM, Ottaviani G, Rossi L, Matturri L (2004) Cytoarchitectural organization of the Parabrachial/Kölliker-Fuse complex in man. Brain Dev 26:316–320

137. Lavezzi AM, Ottaviani G, Rossi L, Matturri L (2004) Hypoplasia of the parabrachial/Kölliker-Fuse complex in perinatal death. Biol Neonate 86:92–97

138. Lavezzi AM, Ottaviani G, Matturri L (2005) Adverse effects of prenatal tobacco smoke exposure on biological parameters of the developing brainstem. Neurobiol Dis 20:601–607

139. Lavezzi AM, Ottaviani G, Matturri L (2005) Biology of the smooth muscle cells in human atherosclerosis. APMIS 113:112–121

140. Lavezzi AM, Ottaviani G, Mauri M, Terni L, Matturri L (2005) Involvement of the EN-2 gene in normal and abnormal development of the human arcuate nucleus. Int J Exp Pathol 86:25–31

141. Lavezzi AM, Ottaviani G, Mingrone R, Matturri L (2005) Analysis of the human locus coeruleus in perinatal and infant sudden unexplained deaths. Possible role of the cigarette smoking in the development of this nucleus. Brain Res Dev Brain Res 154:71–80

142. Lavezzi AM, Ottaviani G, Mauri M, Matturri L (2006) Alterations of biological features of the cerebellum in sudden perinatal and infant death. Curr Mol Med 6:429–435

143. Lavezzi AM, Ottaviani G, Terni L, Matturri L (2006) Histological and biological developmen-

tal characterization of the human cerebellar cortex. Int J Dev Neurosci 24:365–371

144. Lie JT, Rosenberg HS, Erickson EE (1976) Histopathology of the conduction system in the sudden infant death syndrome. Circulation 53:3–8

145. Lobban CD (1995) The oxygen-conserving dive reflex re-examined as the principal contributory factor in the sudden infant death. Med Hypotheses 44:273–277

146. Lonsdale D (2001) Sudden infant death syndrome requires genetic predisposition, some form of stress and marginal malnutrition. Med Hypotheses 57:382–386

147. Luna LG (1973) Manual of histologic staining methods of the Armed Force Institute of Pathology, 3rd edn. Mc Graw-Hill, New York

148. Lundemose JB, Gregerson N, Kolvara S, Pederson BN, Gregersen M, Helweg-Larsen K, Simonsen J (1993) The frequency of a disease-causing point mutation in the gene coding for medium-chain acyl-CoA dehydrogenase in sudden infant death syndrome. Acta Paediatr 82:544–546

149. Malloy MH, Hoffman HJ (1995) Prematurity, sudden infant death syndrome, and age at death. Pediatrics 96:464–471

150. Marino TA, Kane BM (1985) Cardiac atrioventricular junctional tissues in hearts from infants who died suddenly. J Am Coll Cardiol 5:1178–1184

151. Marino TA, Haldar S, Williamson EC, Beaverson K, Walter RA, Marino DR, Beatty C, Lipson KE (1991) Proliferating cell nuclear antigen in developing and adult rat cardiac muscle cells. Circ Res 69:1353–1360

152. Markestad T, Skadberg B, Hordvik E, Morild I, Irgens LM (1995) Sleeping position and sudden infant death syndrome (SIDS): effect of an intervention program to avoid prone sleeping. Acta Paediatr 84:375–378

153. Martinez FD (1991) Sudden infant death syndrome and small airway occlusion: facts and hypothesis. Pediatrics 87:190–198

154. Massing GK, James TN (1976) Anatomical configuration of the His bundle and bundle branches in the human heart. Circulation 53:609–621

155. Matthews TG (1992) The autonomic nervous system: a role in sudden infant death syndrome. Arch Dis Child 67:654–656

156. Matturri L, Rossi L (1994) Tecniche e criteri anatomo-patologici e medico-legali nella diagnostica della morte improvvisa cardiaca. Pathologica 86:430–451

157. Matturri L, Ghidoni P, Rossi L (1986) Miocellule specifiche senoatriali extranodali nella cresta terminale. G Ital Cardiol 16:947–954

158. Matturri L, Nappo A, Varesi C, Martini I, Rossi L (1997) Dualismo del nodo atrioventricolare per la presenza del nodo del seno coronarico di Zahn in un caso di morte improvvisa del lattante (SIDS). Riv Ital Pediatr 23:130–133

159. Matturri L, Ottaviani G, Biondo B, Ramos SG, Rossi L (1998) Discrete T-lymphocytic leptomeningitis of the ventral medullary surface in a case of sudden unexpected infant death. Adv Clin Path 2:313–316

160. Matturri L, Ottaviani G, Rossi L (1999) Sudden and unexpected infant death due to an hemangioendothelioma located in the medulla oblongata. Adv Clin Path 3:29–33

161. Matturri L, Ottaviani G, Ramos SG, Rossi L (2000) Sudden infant death syndrome (SIDS). a study of cardiac conduction system. Cardiovasc Pathol 9:137–145

162. Matturri L, Ottaviani G, Lavezzi AM, Turconi P, Cazzullo A, Rossi L (2001) Expression of apoptosis and proliferating cell nuclear antigen (PCNA) in the cardiac conduction system of crib death (SIDS). Adv Clin Path 5:79–86

163. Matturri L, Biondo B, Suàrez-Mier MP, Rossi L (2002) Brain stem lesions in the sudden infant death syndrome: variability in the hypoplasia of the arcuate nucleus. Acta Neuropathol (Berl) 194:12–20

164. Matturri L, Lavezzi AM, Ottaviani G, Alfonsi G, Crippa M, Rossi L (2002) Anatomo-pathological techniques for the study of brainstem in sudden infant death syndrome (SIDS) and unexpected late fetal stillbirth. In: Proceedings of the 7th SIDS International Conference, Florence, Italy, pp 131–132

165. Matturri L, Lavezzi AM, Ottaviani G, Rossi L (2002) Anatomia patologica della sindrome della morte improvvisa del lattante (SIDS) e della morte inaspettata del feto. In: Proceedings of the National Symposium "Sudden Infant Death Syndrome (SIDS) and Sudden Unexplained Intrauterine Death", Milan, Italy, pp 13–23

166. Matturri L, Lavezzi AM, Rossi L (2002) Proposal to modify the definition of SIDS, with regard to the post-mortem exam. In: Proceedings of the 7th International Conference on SIDS, Florence, Italy, p 103

167. Matturri L, Minoli I, Lavezzi AM, Cappellini A, Ramos S, Rossi L (2002) Hypoplasia of medullary arcuate nucleus in unexpected late fetal death (stillborn infants): a pathological study. Pediatrics 109:E43

168. Matturri L, Ottaviani G, Ballabio G, Lavezzi AM (2002) Medullary arcuate nucleus' cellular differentiation in SIDS and unexpected late fetal stillbirth cases. In: Proceedings of the 7th SIDS International Conference. Florence, Italy, p 135

169. Matturri L, Ottaviani G, Biondo B, Rossi L (2002) Sudden infant death syndrome (SIDS): associated alterations of the cardiac conduction system and brainstem. In: Proceedings of the 7th International Conference on SIDS, Florence, Italy, p 133

170. Matturri L, Ottaviani G, Rossi L (2002) Should overdone external cardiac massage in infants dying of SIDS be discouraged? In: Proceedings of the 7th International Conference on SIDS, Florence, Italy, p 136

171. Matturri L, Lavezzi AM, Minoli I, Ottaviani G, Cappellini A, Rubino B, Rossi L (2003) Association between pulmonary hypoplasia and hypoplasia of arcuate nucleus in stillbirth. J Perinatol 23:328–332

172. Matturri L, Lavezzi AM, Ottaviani G, Rossi L (2003) Intimal preatherosclerotic thickening of the coronary arteries in human fetuses of smoker mothers. J Thromb Haemost 1:2234–2238

173. Matturri L, Ottaviani G, Rossi L (2003) External cardiac massage in infants. Intensive Care Med 29:1199–1200

174. Matturri L, Ottaviani G, Alfonsi G, Crippa M, Rossi L, Lavezzi AM (2004) Study of the brainstem, particularly the arcuate nucleus, in sudden infant death syndrome (SIDS) and sudden intrauterine unexplained death (SIUD). Am J Forensic Med Pathol 25:44–48

175. Matturri L, Ottaviani G, Corti G, Lavezzi AM (2004) Pathogenesis of early atherosclerotic lesions in infants. Pathol Res Pract 200:403–410

176. Matturri L, Ottaviani G, Lavezzi AM (2004) Autoptic examination in sudden infant death syndrome and sudden intrauterine unexpected death: proposal of a national law. J Matern Fetal Neonatal Med 16 [Suppl 2]:43–45

177. Matturri L, Ottaviani G, Lavezzi AM, Rossi L (2004) Early atherosclerotic lesions of the cardiac conduction system arteries in infants. Cardiovasc Pathol 13:276–281

178. Matturri L, Ottaviani G, Benedetti G, Agosta E, Lavezzi AM (2005) Unexpected perinatal death and sudden infant death syndrome (SIDS): anatomopathologic and legal aspects. Am J Forensic Med Pathol 26:155–160

179. Matturri L, Ottaviani G, Lavezzi AM (2005) Early atherosclerotic lesions in infancy: role of parental cigarette smoking. Virchows Arch 447:74–80

180. Matturri L, Ottaviani G, Lavezzi AM (2005) Sudden infant death triggered by dive reflex. J Clin Pathol 58:77–80

181. Matturri L, Ottaviani G, Lavezzi AM (2005) Techniques and criteria in pathologic and forensic-medical diagnostics in sudden unexpected infant and perinatal death. Am J Clin Pathol 124:259–268

182. Matturri L, Ottaviani G, Lavezzi AM (2005) Unexpected sudden death related to medullary brain lesions. Acta Neuropathol (Berl) 109:554–555

183. Matturri L, Ottaviani G, Lavezzi AM, Grana D, Milei J (2005) Madres fumadoras y aterosclerosis prenatal. Rev Argent Cardiol 73:366–369

184. Matturri L, Ottaviani G, Lavezzi AM, Ramos SG (2005) Peripheral chemoreceptors and sudden infant death syndrome: a wide open problem. Curr Cardiol Rev 1:65–70

185. Matturri L, Ottaviani G, Lavezzi AM (2006) Maternal smoking and sudden infant death syndrome: epidemiological study related to pathology. Virchows Arch 449:697–706

186. Milner AD (1987) Recent theories on the cause of cot death. Br Med J 295:1366–1368
187. Mitchell EA, Scragg L, Clements M (1996) Soft cot mattresses and the sudden infant death syndrome. N Z Med J 109:206–207
188. Mitchell EA, Stewart AW (1997) Gender and the sudden infant death syndrome. New Zealand Cot Death Group. Acta Paediatr 86:854–856
189. Moon HD (1957) Coronary arteries in fetuses, infants and juveniles: Circulation 16:263–267
190. Morpurgo CV, Lavezzi AM, Ottaviani G, Rossi L (2004) Bulbo-spinal pathology and sudden respiratory infant death syndrome. Eur J Anaesthesiol 21:589–593
191. Nachmanoff DB, Panigrahy A, Filiano JJ, Sieeper LA, Valdes-Dapena M, Krous HF, White WF, Kinney HC (1998) Brainstem H3-nicotine receptor binding in the sudden infant death syndrome. J Neuropathol Exp Neurol 57:1018–1025
192. Nattie E, Kinney H (2002) Nicotine, serotonine, and sudden infant death syndrome. Am J Respir Crit Care Med 166:1544–1549
193. Olszewski J, Baxter D (1982) Cytoarchitecture of the human brain stem. Karger, Basel
194. Orenstein SR, Mitchell AA, Ward SD (1993) Concerning the American Academy of Pediatrics recommendation on sleep position for infants. Pediatrics 91:497–499
195. Ottaviani G (2006) Histological observation of the cardiac conduction system in the diagnostics of sudden infant death syndrome (SIDS). "SIDS e ALTE Aggiornamento 2005. Primo Corso Teorico Pratico di Anatomia-Patologica in casi di Sospetta SIDS e di morte inaspettata fetale", 19 October 2005, Parma, Italy. Acta Biomed Ateneo Parmense 77:52
196. Ottaviani G (2006) Histopathological study of the cardiac conduction system in systemic lupus erythematosus. J Postgrad Med 52:10
197. Ottaviani G (2006) How to sample the cardiac conduction system. "SIDS e ALTE Aggiornamento 2005. Primo Corso Teorico Pratico di Anatomia-Patologica in casi di Sospetta SIDS e di morte inaspettata fetale", 19 October 2005, Parma, Italy. Acta Biomed Ateneo Parmense 77:50
198. Ottaviani G, Ramos SG, Matturri L (1997) Defective "resorptive degeneration" of the heart's conduction system and sudden infant death syndrome. Ann Espan Pediatr (Suppl) 92:53
199. Ottaviani G, Goisis M, Ramos SG, Matturri L (1998) Dispersione del tessuto giunzionale e sue conseguenze in un caso di morte improvvisa del lattante. Cardiologia 43:737–739
200. Ottaviani G, Matturri L, Ramos SG, Rossi L (1998) Resorptive degeneration of the heart's conduction system and sudden infant death syndrome: preliminary results. In: Proceedings of the 5th SIDS International Conference, Rouen, France, p 156
201. Ottaviani G, Rossi L, Bondurri A, Ramos SG, Matturri L (1998) Morte improvvisa del lattante: un caso di sdoppiamento del nodo atrio-ventricolare. Riv Ital Pediatr 24:1165–1167
202. Ottaviani G, Lavezzi AM, De Ruberto F, Fichera G, Matturri L (1999) The prognostic value of cell proliferation in colorectal adenomas assessed with tritiated thymidine and anti-proliferating cell nuclear antigen (PCNA). Cancer Detect Prev 23:57–63
203. Ottaviani G, Lavezzi AM, Rossi L, Matturri L (1999) Proliferating cell nuclear antigen (PCNA) and apoptosis in hyperacute and acute myocardial infarction. Eur J Histochem 43:7–14
204. Ottaviani G, Rossi L, Ramos SG, Matturri L (1999) Pathology of the heart and conduction system in a case of sudden death due to a cardiac fibroma in a 6-month-old child. Cardiovasc Pathol 8:109–112
205. Ottaviani G, Rossi L, Varesi C, Ramos SG, Matturri L (1999) Pathology of the cardiac conduction system in sudden infant death syndrome (SIDS): preliminary results. Pediatr Res (Suppl) 45:23A
206. Ottaviani G, James TN, Rossi L, Matturri L (2002) Significance of Mahaim fibers in crib death. In: Proceedings of the 7th SIDS International Conference, Florence, Italy, p 136
207. Ottaviani G, Matturri L, Lavezzi AM, Rossi L, James TN (2002) Postnatal apoptosis of the cardiac conduction system in crib death: preliminary results. In: Proceedings of the 7th SIDS International Conference, Florence, Italy, p 132
208. Ottaviani G, Matturri L, Rossi L, James TN (2002) Crib death: further support for the concept of fatal cardiac electrical instability as the final common pathway. In: Proceedings of the 7th SIDS International Conference, Florence, Italy, p 66

209. Ottaviani G, Rossi L, Matturri L (2002) Histopathology of the cardiac conduction system in a case of metastatic pancreatic ductal adenocarcinoma. Anticancer Res 22:3029–3032

210. Ottaviani G, Matturri L, Rossi L, James TN (2003) Crib death: further support for the concept of fatal cardiac electrical instability as the final common pathway. Int J Cardiol 92:17–26

211. Ottaviani G, Matturri L, Rossi L, Jones D (2003) Sudden death due to lymphomatous infiltration of the cardiac conduction system. Cardiovasc Pathol 12:77–81

212. Ottaviani G, Lavezzi AM, Rossi L, Matturri L (2004) Sudden unexpected death of a term fetus in a anticardiolipin positive mother. Am J Perinatol 21:31–35

213. Ottaviani G, Matturri L, Rossi L, Lavezzi AM, James TN (2004) Multifocal cardiac Purkinje cell tumor in infancy. Europace 6:138–141

214. Ottaviani G, Matturri L, Bruni B, Lavezzi AM (2005) Sudden infant death syndrome "gray zone" disclosed only by a study of the brain stem on serial sections. J Perinat Med 33:165–169

215. Ottaviani G, Rossi L, Matturri L (2005) Myocardial injury attributable to external cardiac massage in infants. Cardiology 1:25–29

216. Ottaviani G, Lavezzi AM, Matturri L (2006) Sudden infant death syndrome (SIDS) shortly after hexavalent vaccination: another pathology in suspected SIDS? Virchows Arch 448:100–104

217. Ottaviani G, Matturri L, Mingrone R, Lavezzi AM (2006) Hypoplasia and neuronal immaturity of the hypoglossal nucleus in sudden infant death. J Clin Pathol 59:497–500

218. Pinholster G (1995) Multiple "SIDS" case ruled murder. Science 268:494

219. Ponsonby AL, Dwyer T, Gibbson LE, Cochrane JA, Jones ME, McCall MJ (1992) Thermal environment and sudden infant death syndrome: case-control study. BMJ 304:277–282

220. Presti C (1994) Metodiche immunoistochimiche per la dimostrazione della periferia nervosa intracardiaca. Pathologica 86:443–449

221. Priori SG, Bloise R, Crotti L (2001) The long QT syndrome. Europace 3:16–27

222. Ramos SG, Matturri L, Biondo B, Ottaviani G, Rossi L (1998) Hyperplasia of the aorticopulmonary paraganglia: a new insight into the pathogenesis of sudden infant death syndrome? Cardiologia 43:953–958

223. Ramos SG, Matturri L, Ottaviani G, Rossi L (1998) Maternal smoking and aorticopulmonary paraganglia in sudden infant death syndrome. In: Proceedings of the 5th SIDS International Conference, Rouen, France, p 169

224. Ramos SG, Ottaviani G, Biondo B, Rossi L, Matturri L (1999) Hyperplasia of the aortico-pulmonary paraganglia in infants dying of SIDS: further supports for the cardiorespiratory hypothesis. In: Proceedings of the International Symposium on SIDS and Lombardy Region project for the reduction of the risk for sudden infant death and unexplained intrauterine death, Milan, Italy, pp 117–128

225. Raring RH (1975) Crib death. Exposition Press, New York

226. Robertson JH (1960) The significance of intimal thickening in the arteries of the newborn. Arch Dis Child 35:588–590

227. Rossi L (1969) Histopathologic features of cardiac arrhythmias. Casa Editrice Ambrosiana, Milan

228. Rossi L (1975) A histological survey of pre-excitation syndrome and related arrhythmias. G Ital Cardiol 5:816–828

229. Rossi L (1978) Intramural ramification of the left bundle branch. Am Heart J 96:271–272

230. Rossi L (1978) "Salvage the pacemaker" at autopsy. Am Heart J 95:540–541

231. Rossi L (1983) The pathologic basis of cardiac arrhythmias. Cardiol Clin 1:13–17

232. Rossi L (1998) Histopathology of the cardiac conduction system in the problem of arrhythmogenic SIDS. In: Proceedings of the 18th International Symposium on Neonatal Intensive Care, Milan, Italy, p 75

233. Rossi L (1999) Bulbo-spinal pathology in neurocardiac sudden death of adults: a prognostic approach to a neglected problem. Int J Legal Med 112:83–90

234. Rossi L, Matturri L (1985) Histopathology of aortocoronary glomera: modern anatomo-clini-

cal approach to the understanding of cardiocirculatory disorders. G Ital Cardiol 15:718–724

235. Rossi L, Matturri L (1988) His bundle haematoma and external cardiac massage: histopathological findings. Br Heart J 59:586–587

236. Rossi L, Matturri L (1990) Clinicopathological approach to cardiac arrhythmias. A color atlas. Centro Scientifico Torinese, Turin

237. Rossi L, Matturri L (1991) Anatomohistological features of sudden infant death. New Trends Arrhyt 6:135–142

238. Rossi L, Matturri L (1995) Anatomo-histological features of the heart's conduction system and innervation in SIDS. In: Rognum TO (ed) Sudden infant death syndrome: new trends in the nineties. Scandinavian University Press, Oslo, pp 207–212

239. Rossi L, Matturri L (1995) Cardiac conduction and nervous system in health disease and sudden death: an anatomoclinical overview. Osp Maggiore 89:239–257

240. Rossi L, Matturri L (1998) Neuronal degeneration localized in the thoracic spinal cord sympathetic center in a case with prolonged QT interval. G Ital Cardiol (Suppl) 28:535–537

241. Rossi L, Thiene G (1983) Arrhythmologic pathology of sudden cardiac death. Casa Editrice Ambrosiana, Milan

242. Rossi L, Knippel M, Taccardi B (1975) Histological findings, His bundle recordings and body-surface potential mappings in a case of Wolff-Parkinson-White syndrome. An anatomoclinical comparison. Cardiology 60:265–279

243. Rossi L, Thiene G, Knippel M (1978) A case of surgically corrected Wolff-Parkinson-White syndrome: clinical and histological data. Br Heart J 40:581–585

244. Rossi L, Piffer R, Turolla E, Frigerio B, Coumel P, James TN (1985) Multifocal purkinje-like tumor of the heart. Occurrence with other anatomic abnormalities in the atrioventricular junction of an infant with junctional tachycardia, Lown-Ganong-Levine syndrome, and sudden death. Chest 87:340–345

245. Rossi L, Matturri L, Lotto A (1988) Cardiac conduction blocks and pacemaking. An anatomoclinical color atlas. Clas International, Brescia

246. Rossi L, Pozzato R, Matturri L (1991) L'anatomia patologica della morte cardiaca oggi. Riv Ital Med Leg 13:93–110

247. Rossi L, Matturri L, Ottaviani G (2002) Arrhythmogenic sudden death in the modern setting SIDS. An overview. In: Proceedings of the 7th International Conference on SIDS, Florence, Italy, p 153

248. Rossi L, Matturri L, Ottaviani G (2002) Sudden unexpected death of a term fetus with maternal infant anti-cardiolipin antibodies. A case report. In: Proceedings of the 7th International Conference on SIDS, Florence, Italy, p 137

249. Rumyantsev PP (1977) Interrelations of the proliferation and differentiation processes during cardiac myogenesis and regeneration. Int Rev Cytol 51:187–273

250. Ruth G (1994) The changing epidemiology of SIDS. Arch Dis Child 70:445–449

251. Saunders JW (1966) Death in embryonic systems. Science 154:604–612

252. Sawczenko A, Fleming PJ (1996) Thermal stress, sleeping position, and the sudden infant death syndrome. Sleep 19:267–270

253. Schauer GM, Kalousek DK, Magel JF (1992) Genetic causes of stillbirth. Semin Perinatol 16:341–351

254. Schwartz PJ, Stramba-Badiale M, Segantini A, Austoni P, Bosi G, Giorgetti RR, Grancini F, Marini ED, Perticone F, Rositi D, Salice P (1998) Prolongation of the QT interval and the sudden infant death syndrome. N Engl J Med 338:1709–1714

255. Schwartz PJ, Priori SG, Dumaine R, Napolitano C, Antzelevitch C, Stramba-Badiale M, Richard TA, Berti MR, Bloise R (2000) A molecular link between the sudden infant death syndrome and the long-QT syndrome. N Engl J Med 343:262–267

256. Sciacca A, Mascagni MT, De Andreis M (1958) Morphological contribution to the knowledge of pathogenesis of branch block; serial histological study and reconstruction of His-Tawara bundle in man. Cuore Circ 42:321–345

257. Scragg R, Mitchell EA, Taylor BJ, Stewart AW, Ford RPK, Thompson JMD, Allen EM, Becroft

DMO (1993) Bed sharing, smoking and alcohol in the sudden infant death syndrome. BMJ 307:1312–1318

258. Shannon DC, Kelly DH (1982) SIDS and near-SIDS (first of two parts). N Engl J Med 306:959–965

259. Shannon DC, Kelly DH (1982) SIDS and near-SIDS (second of two parts). N Engl J Med 306:1022–1028

260. Southall DP, Arrowsmith WA, Stebbins V, Alexander JR (1986) QT interval measurements before sudden infant death syndrome. Arch Dis Child 61:327–333

261. Spiers PS, Onstad L, Guntheroth WG (1996) Negative effect of a short interpregnancy interval on birth weight following loss of an infant to sudden infant death syndrome. Am J Epidemiol 143:1137–1141

262. Spinner S, Gibson E, Wrobel H, Spitzer AR (1995) Recent advantages in home infant apnea monitoring. Neonatal Netw 14:39–46

263. Suàrez-Mier MP, Aguilera B (1998) Histopathology of the conduction system in sudden infant death. Forensic Sci Int 93:143–154

264. Suàrez-Mier MP, Gamallo C (1998) Atrioventricular node fetal dispersion and His fragmentation of the cardiac conduction system in sudden cardiac death. J Am Coll Cardiol 32:1885–1890

265. Tawara S (1906) Das Reizleitungssystem des Sàugetierherzens. G. Fisher, Jena

266. Taylor A (1996) Antimony, cot mattresses, and SIDS. Lancet 347:616

267. Thiene G (1988) Problems in the interpretation of cardiac pathology in reference to SIDS. Ann N Y Acad Sci 533:191–199

268. Topaz O, Castellanos A, Grobman LR, Myerburg RJ (1988) The role of arrhythmogenic auditory stimuli in sudden cardiac death. Am Heart J 116:222–226

269. Valdès-Dapena M (1985) Are some crib deaths sudden cardiac deaths? J Am Coll Cardiol 5 (6 Suppl):113B–117B

270. Valdés-Dapena M, Gilbert-Barness E (2002) Cardiovascular causes for sudden infant death. Pediatr Pathol Mol Med 21:195–211

271. Valdés-Dapena M, Huff D (1983) Perinatal autopsy manual. Armed Forces Institute of Pathology, Washington DC

272. Valdés-Dapena MA, Greene M, Basavanand N, Catherman R, Truex RC (1973) The myocardial conduction system in sudden death in infancy. N Engl J Med 289:1179–1180

273. Valdès-Dapena M, McFreeley PA, Hoffman HJ, Damus KH, Franciosi RR, Allison DJ, Jones M, Hunter JC (1993) Histopathology atlas for the sudden infant death syndrome. Armed Forces Institute of Pathology, Washington DC

274. Van Baarlen J, Schuurman HJ, Huber J (1988) Acute thymus involution in infancy and childhood: a reliable marker for duration of acute illness. Hum Pathol 19:1155–1160

275. Vance JC, Boyle FM, Najman JM, Thearle MJ (2002) Couple distress after sudden infant or perinatal death: a 30-month follow up. J Paediatr Child Health 38:368–372

276. Viskin S, Fish R, Roth A, Schwartz PJ, Belhassen B (2000) QT or not QT? N Engl J Med 343:352–356

277. Waldo AL, James TN (1973) A retrospective look at A-V nodal rhythms (A Zahn). Circulation 47:222–224

278. Weller U, Jorch G (1993) Current percentile curves for body weight, body length and head circumference of newborn infants after the 25th week of pregnancy. Monatsschr Kinderheilkd 141:665–669

279. Widdicombe JG, Tatar M (1988) Upper airway reflex control. Ann N Y Acad Sci 533:252–261

280. Willinger M, James LS, Catz C (1991) Defining the sudden infant death syndrome (SIDS): deliberations of an expert panel convened by the National Institute of Child Health Development. Pediatr Pathol 11:677–684

281. Willinger M, Hoffman HJ, Hartford RB (1994) Infant sleep position and risk for sudden infant death syndrome: report of meeting held January 13 and 14, 1994, National Institutes of Health, Bethesda, MD. Pediatrics 93:814–819

282. Wolff GS, Han J, Curran G (1978) Wolff-Parkinson-White syndrome in the neonate. Am J Cardiol 41:559–563
283. World Health Organization (2007) World Health Assembly, WHA55 – 13–18 May 2002. http://www.who.int/gb/e/e_wha55.html. Cited 1 Feb 2007
284. Wren C (1998) Mechanism of fetal tachycardia. Heart 79:536–539
285. Zahn A (1912) Experimentelle untersuchungen über die reizbildung im atrioventrikularnoten und sinus coronarius. Zentralbl Physiol 26:495
286. Zec N, Filiano JJ, Kinney HC (1997) Anatomic relationship of the human arcuate nucleus of the medulla: a Dil-labeling study. J Neuropathol Exp Neurol 56:509–522

Subject Index